The Scandalous Neglect of Children's Mental Health

What Schools Can Do

James M. Kauffman
and Jeanmarie Badar

Routledge
Taylor & Francis Group

NEW YORK AND LONDON

First published 2018
by Routledge
711 Third Avenue, New York, NY 10017

and by Routledge
2 Park Square, Milton Park, Abingdon, Oxon, OX14 4RN

Routledge is an imprint of the Taylor & Francis Group, an informa business

© 2018 Taylor & Francis

Library of Congress Cataloging-in-Publication Data
A catalog record for this book has been requested

ISBN: 978-0-8153-4893-1 (hbk)
ISBN: 978-0-8153-4895-5 (pbk)
ISBN: 978-1-351-16580-8 (ebk)

Typeset in Palatino
by Apex CoVantage, LLC

The Scandalous Neglect of Children's Mental Health

The Scandalous Neglect of Children's Mental Health: What Schools Can Do makes the case that children with mental health needs are under-identified and under-served by schools and other agencies. After reading this brief but powerful book, you will better understand the need for expanded services for children in schools and communities. The risks and benefits of treatment, especially early intervention, are discussed and guidelines for action by teachers, parents, and others are provided. The sad fact is that many people do not understand that most young people with mental health needs never receive any treatment of any kind and most of those who receive any treatment at all receive those services only in schools.

James M. Kauffman is Professor Emeritus of Education at the Curry School of Education at the University of Virginia. He was the William Clay Parrish Professor of Education 1992–1994, the Charles S. Robb Professor of Education 1999–2003, and received the Outstanding Faculty Award from the Curry School of Education in 1997. He received the Research Award, Council for Exceptional Children in 1994 and the Outstanding Leadership Award, Council for Children with Behavioral Disorders in 2002.

Jeanmarie Badar is Instructional Assistant in second-grade classrooms in the Charlottesville City Schools. She was a special education teacher for 25 years and served on the faculty of James Madison University. She completed her Master's degree in special education at Kent State University (KSU) and received her Ph.D. from the University of Virginia. The Badar/Kauffman endowed Conference on Contemporary Issues in Special Education at KSU was named in her honor. She is co-author with James M. Kauffman, Daniel P. Hallahan, and Paige C. Pullen of another Routledge book published in 2018, the second edition of *Special Education: What It Is and Why We Need It*.

Dedicated to the Loving Memories of Our Late Spouses
Patricia L. Pullen
Steven G. Bantz

And to the Loving Memory of Jeanmarie Badar's Late Father
Lawrence J. Badar

Gifted Teachers All

Contents

Meet the Authors

We describe individually some of our relevant experiences that have influenced what we've written. This experience includes not only our work with children and teachers but also our training as educators in both general and special education and our familiarity with mental health issues and services.

James M. Kauffman

I began teaching general education in a public school in 1962. However, among my early employment was teaching emotionally disturbed children and adolescents in a private psychiatric residential treatment center. Children with emotional and behavioral problems may be called by a variety of legitimate labels. Among them are "emotionally disturbed," "mentally ill," "behaviorally disordered," or "children with emotional and behavioral disorders." The labels don't matter much, but the difficulties these children and their families and their teachers experience matter a lot. The children I taught in a residential treatment center were called "emotionally disturbed." In my work in the treatment center, I had frequent contact with child psychiatrists and psychologists as well as other teachers.

Like most people, I didn't realize when I began teaching that most children with mental health needs are in regular public schools, going to regular classes. Often, they have been driving their teachers to distraction. Too often, their problems are neglected or are met with counterproductive responses from others. I eventually became a teacher of both general and special education in public schools, and since then I have studied the problems and treatments of children and youth with mental health needs as well as the typical behavior of children and youth. I have trained and supervised teachers in a variety of school settings, been a consultant to private and public schools and institutions, and engaged in considerable research and publication involving exceptional children. I have studied and written about those having mental health needs as well as those having a variety of disabilities and special gifts or talents. Some of the children I have studied have had special mental health needs as well as other exceptionalities.

I am an educator by training and experience, not a psychologist or psychiatrist. Nevertheless, a substantial proportion of my training and experience has involved study of the literatures, concepts, and practices of psychology and psychiatry. Perhaps it is fair to say that I am an educator with more than the typical grounding in children's mental health problems and what to do about them. Eventually, I earned my Doctor of Education degree in special education at the University of Kansas, where my emphasis was on educating children with emotional and behavioral disorders (EBD).

The fact is that most people who need mental health services don't get them. Psychologists and psychiatrists know this. I know this as an educator with special concerns for children and youths with emotional and behavioral problems. My research and writing have been about children in schools, not adults. Jeanmarie and I hope to promote kinder and more effective treatment of children whose behavior and/or emotional development has gone off the tracks.

I'm deeply indebted to my late mentor, Richard J. Whelan, Ed.D., an extraordinary teacher, researcher, writer, speaker, administrator, and distinguished professor of special education, child development, and pediatrics and lecturer in psychiatry at the University of Kansas. He also served in what is now the U.S. Department of Education, Office of Special Education Programs. Early in his career, he became principal of the Southard School (the Children's Division of the Menninger Psychiatric Clinic), where he introduced me to the field of special education for children with mental health difficulties.

Jeanmarie Badar

I was a special education teacher for 25 years, mostly working with students with serious mental health problems. I remember feeling overwhelmed and underprepared to work with this population, even though my undergraduate program at Boston College was otherwise quite good. My very first teaching job was in a small suburban public school district near Cleveland, where I was tasked with creating a brand-new program for K–3 students with severe behavior handicaps

(SBH). Fortunately for me, I had help from a special education consultant who worked with teachers in several school districts. Not only did she take me step-by-step through the process of setting up a classroom management system and instructional plan, she visited at least weekly to offer hands-on support and problem-solving. Early on, she arranged for me to visit other well-established classes for students with SBH and consult with experienced teachers at the Positive Education Program (PEP), which operates several day treatment centers in Ohio under the auspices of the Cuyahoga County School District and the Cuyahoga County Board of Mental Health. For my second year of teaching, I pursued a job with PEP, where I worked for the next three years. To this day, I credit the people at PEP for giving me the foundational knowledge and skills to become a really good teacher of children with emotional and behavioral disabilities (EBD). I learned the importance of appropriate instruction, first and foremost, in preventing problem behavior. I became skilled at developing classroom rules, routines, and procedures that helped students feel safe and competent. I learned how to build and maintain trusting relationships with my students and how to ensure that I was teaching and recognizing desirable behaviors more than correcting misbehavior. And I became an expert at creating a classroom community that promoted kindness, compassion, and belonging. Most importantly, my years with PEP cemented my commitment to students with EBD for the remainder of my teaching career.

From there, I continued to teach students with EBD in various public schools (my husband's job as an engineer required us to move around a bit for the first decade of our marriage), and I spent two years living and teaching in Singapore, which was quite an adventure! Over the years, however, I began to notice some disturbing trends in special education: eligibility teams were becoming more and more reluctant to identify a child as having EBD or mental health problems; and placement decisions seemed to be based not so much on a student's individual needs but mostly on a school's or administrator's belief in the inclusion of students with disabilities in general education. I saw many of the instructional and behavior management strategies and tools I had learned become unavailable to me because my "self-contained" classroom now resembled a poorly designed resource room, with students coming and going all day long, everyone following different schedules and dealing with a different set of teachers. My role was becoming one of "putting out fires" all day long rather than helping kids learn the academic and behavioral skills they needed to succeed in school. This is where I experienced the "scandalous neglect" we speak of in this book.

I taught for a total of 25 years, during which time I earned my Master's degree and Ph.D. in Special Education with a focus on EBD. I worked with some very forward-looking teachers and administrators who recognized the need to provide more appropriate, intensive services for students with mental health problems. Eventually, however, I left special education for general education, in large part because I felt like I was not getting students with mental health problems the kind of help they needed. I hope that this little book may help others recognize how our schools can and should become better at preventing, recognizing, and treating mental health problems of children and youth.

Preface

This little book is a simple, direct explanation of our society's seeming unwillingness to address the mental health needs of children. Its audience is anyone eager to learn about how badly children and youth with mental health problems are treated in our society and what they can do about it.

Unawareness of the mental health needs of our children and youth by many in our society is common. The mental health problems of youngsters are seldom treated in any way whatsoever or are treated ineffectively, in part because of the misunderstanding or disinterest of the public. This is not to say that the mental health needs of adults are recognized and treated any better. In fact, they aren't by much, if at all. Streets and jails are where you'll find most adults with severe mental illness these days, not hospitals or places of refuge. And the needs of many young people with mental health problems are often neglected until they come to the attention of the juvenile justice system and are incarcerated. Treatment of adults is something we leave to others to write about; we focus on children.

We do understand that the mental health problems of most adults started when they were children and have gone unrecognized and untreated for years. That's one of the reasons we've written this little book. We also understand the central role of schooling in the lives of children. Other than parents, teachers are the people most likely to know of a child's mental health problems. In fact, teachers may observe children's mental health difficulties in school when the problems are not apparent at home. Teachers are in a particularly good position to become first responders to these problems.

Acknowledgements

Editor Alex Masulis gave us support for this project, as did many working to see the booklet through production.

Besides those working on development of the manuscript and book at Routledge, we acknowledge with thanks the encouragement of many colleagues, friends, and former students, all too numerous to name. We are especially grateful to those associated with the Midwest Symposium for Leadership in Behavior Disorders (MSLBD; see MSLBD.org) and Teacher Educators for Children with Behavior Disorders (TECBD; see education.asu.edu/annual-tecbd-conference. A conference on autism has been named in honor of the late Rich Simpson, Ed.D., one of the founders of MSLBD, a dear friend and colleague who died in 2017.).

Among our friends and colleagues frequently attending and presenting research at these conferences are special educator and psychologist Steven R. Forness, Ed.D. and child/adolescent psychiatrist Richard E. (Dick) Mattison, M.D. For many years, Steve was a psychologist at and principal of the Neuropsychiatric Institute School (the school in the NPI hospital of UCLA). Dr. Mattison, now at Pennsylvania State University's College of Medicine, Hershey, obtained his training in child and adolescent psychiatry at UCLA. He specializes in the role of schools and teachers in children's mental health. The work of both Steve and Dick has been particularly important in shaping our thinking about children's mental health and the important role schools can play in addressing youngsters' problems.

1

The Scandal

Scandal is a very strong word, often misused to describe something merely disliked. In fact, just about anything someone thinks shouldn't have been allowed to happen or should have been done but wasn't done can be described, often wrongly, as a scandal. But an actual scandal is something truly shameful that brings dishonor, something that causes or *should* cause public outrage.

American society's failure to recognize and treat children and youth with mental health problems appropriately is outrageous. In fact, we could say it's a *real* scandal. But it's a scandal lots of people don't know about—or they do know about it but deny it or dismiss it as not really important. Some people recognize it as a bad situation but conclude there isn't much we can do about it, which isn't so. Schools can do a lot to address the scandal. But schools alone are not enough.

At least three journalists—Pete Earley, Ron Powers, and Judith Warner—have written poignantly about how people in the general public, including too many educators, have many wrong ideas about problems of behavior and mental health.[1] Earley wrote about the difficulty of getting mental health services for his son and others who are seriously mentally ill. Powers, the parent of two sons with mental health needs, one of whom committed suicide, wrote about how little people seem to care about others with mental health needs. Like

Earley, Powers used the colloquialism "crazy" in referring to mental illness. Not everyone with a serious mental health problem is considered "crazy." Warner wrote about how lots of people believe that youngsters with serious emotional or behavioral problems are identified for no good reason. People may mistakenly believe that difficulties like attention deficit hyperactivity disorder (ADHD) are minor, or believe that kids with such problems typically get undeserved attention, or too much treatment, or too often are medicated.

People often suggest that most children with ADHD or other problems at school just need shaming or stern discipline or physical punishment, ways of reacting to children's behavior that usually make the problems worse. Misunderstanding and mistreatment of children with mental health problems are common in both communities and schools. The fact is that many problems related to mental health are often first noticed in schools, and teachers are therefore in a particularly good position to recognize the scandal and do something about it.

> The fact is that many problems related to mental health are often first noticed in schools, and teachers are therefore in a particularly good position to recognize the scandal and do something about it.

A true scandal is like a low-grade fever, a clear sign that something's wrong and is going to get worse if it isn't dealt with appropriately. The topic of this book is a relatively unknown scandal that doesn't cause much anger in the general public because it's so well disguised. Misinformation is repeated so often, or a false impression is created so well and made so seductive, that most people believe something untrue. They believe things that truly qualify as "fake news."

Too many people don't care about children's mental health. They are ignorant of the facts or wish them away. They think that kids are typically rushed to treatment for minor or imaginary problems, the equivalent of getting overly concerned about the sniffles or giving hypochondriacs attention for their fantasies. Or they don't seem to realize that behavior like that of presidential candidate and later President Donald Trump is indicative of a mental disorder. Some people see Trump's suggestions of violence and torture; his bullying, mocking, and belittling of others; his lack of empathy for fellow human beings; his refusal to apologize or take responsibility for his statements or actions; his mendacity, blaming others for his mistakes or misdeeds; racism, sexism, xenophobia, braggadocio, denial of reality, and self-aggrandizement as normal rather than hideously disturbed.[2] Some people say that Trump's supporters, though, are normal, even if Trump isn't. But, even if most of his supporters are mentally and behaviorally normal, that does not mean President Trump's behavior is normal or should be "normalized" or seen as a model for anyone, child or adult.

Many Americans seem not to recognize some forms of mental illness when they see them, and this unwillingness to see aberrant behavior for what it is, particularly when it is antisocial conduct, contributes to the scandalous neglect of young people's as well as adults' mental health needs. In fact, many individuals in positions of power and authority have chosen to ignore, excuse, or further enable and abet Mr. Trump's verbal and nonverbal behavior. They fail to point out the unacceptability of public displays of emotional ill health, unpredictability, and intellectual instability. In doing so, they likely encourage imitation of unacceptable behavior by youngsters. Agnosticism regarding emotional and behavioral aberrance in high-profile leaders does not suggest timely recognition of the mental health needs of children and youth.[3]

We hasten to add that *most individuals with mental health needs are not dangerous.* Dangerousness is heightened by two things: (1) antisocial behavior, especially aggression and extreme social withdrawal, both of which may be indicated by verbal or physical behavior or a combination of them, and (2) an individual's ability to coerce or harm others, such that the greater the person's sphere of influence, the greater the danger. That is, danger may be confined to parents, siblings, or relatively few others if the person's power over others is relatively low; but the danger is magnified by higher executive authority and greater power over others.

Children may be extremely antisocial, but they seldom have much actual power over others. However, their mental health issues are seldom addressed until those issues have become extreme. Children

> Many Americans seem not to recognize some forms of mental illness when they see them, and this unwillingness to see aberrant behavior for what it is, particularly when it is antisocial conduct, contributes to the scandalous neglect of young people's as well as adults' mental health needs.

experience precisely the opposite of easy access to mental health care. Kids and their parents typically endure horrible problems that aren't addressed for years, if ever.

Clever politicians encourage the misperception of what's scandalous and say we can't afford to deal with such problems now anyway—or offer the opinion that the problem is lack of moral fiber or strength of kids and their families. Or they may tell us, sure, we need better mental health services—but then skirt the issue of cost and never talk about what actually needs to be done. Calls for attention to mental health issues of adults or children are easy, popular, and politically advantageous, particularly after mass shootings, but appropriate action and needed funding are difficult and seldom provided. The real scandal is disguised by evasion and misinformation, which are indefensible on rational as well as moral grounds. But the wrong impression, the evasion and the misinformation, seem to "work," in that they convince the general public to believe a fiction and ignore the truth.

Part of the smoke screen that hides the real scandal has to do with labels. So, we digress somewhat here to address some problems of terminology. Most people don't understand that the real scandal in both mental health and special education is the neglect of children who need help in their homes, communities, and schools. The differences between mental illness and the federal special education category called "emotional disturbance" are important. In some ways, the differences and similarities are confusing, and we discuss the differences and the overlap between them further in Chapter 3. Suffice it to say at this point that they are overlapping and that both mental health (or psychological) services and special education for children and youths with emotional/behavioral disorders or problems are important and that both are characterized by scandalous neglect.[4]

The American Psychiatric Association has its own terminology and acronyms for various forms of mental illness, as we mention below. Children who have mental health problems or need special supports in school because of emotional or behavioral disabilities have attracted many different labels and much confusing terminology. States vary in the terminology they use to designate students falling into various special education categories. Many of these students need special psychological/psychiatric and educational supports, and these supports are often not provided, especially not in schools. For example, an investigation into special education in Chicago public schools found not only that special education funding was reduced in most categories at the expense of students' welfare, but that the largest cuts in services related to special education were in psychological support.[5]

Children with mental health problems are often considered in schools to have "emotional and behavioral disorders" (EBD) or "emotional disturbance" (ED).[6] People may wonder what distinguishes "emotional" from "behavioral," "disturbance" from "disorder," or even divert attention to the conjunctions "and" and "or." In our opinion, these linguistic quibbles have no merit in distinguishing one group of children from another or making better sense of the problem. We should not get hung up on these issues about labels.

Then there are those who don't want to label a child or the child's problems in any way. Well … just try talking about something without saying what it is—using a word (label) for it! And then there are people who want to label the problem or the service, just not the individual. But, if you think about it a little, you'll see that, first, people are always labeled by their special problems; second, people are always labeled by the services they get. And there are those who want to use some euphemism such as "challenged" to avoid social stigma associated with other words. But a euphemism like "challenged" is useless unless its meaning is fudged, simply because everybody faces challenges. "Challenged" and other euphemisms make humorists' careers, because when people figure out how the word is being used they tend to laugh at the clumsy attempt to avoid a reality. We can't do away with labels or avoid labeling kids except by *not talking about* their problems or the services they get, even if we talk only in "code." Worry about labels is mostly a diversion, a distraction from recognizing and dealing with problems. Certainly, we should avoid "street language" and epithets, but not the language (labels) of professionals.

We might also use terms associated with psychiatry, psychology, community mental health services, or special education such as "conduct disorder" (CD), "obsessive-compulsive disorder" (OCD), "oppositional defiant

> We can't do away with labels or avoid labeling kids except by not talking about their problems or the services they get, even if we talk only in "code." Worry about labels is mostly a diversion, a distraction from recognizing and dealing with problems.

disorder" (ODD), "attention deficit hyperactivity disorder" (ADHD), and many others. Terms like these are used in the *Diagnostic and Statistical Manual* of the American Psychiatric Association (often referred to simply as the DSM). These labels may be important for teachers and parents to understand when talking about particular individuals. Terms such as these may convey important information about the nature of a problem and its treatment. However, they must be explained appropriately to teachers and parents.[7]

But, back to the children and youth who are the focus of what we consider a real scandal. Who are we talking about? Not just those in the federal special education category of "emotional disturbance" under the federal law named in 2004 as *The Individuals with Disabilities Education Improvement Act* (originally enacted by Congress in 1975 and better known today as the IDEA). We do focus on those who might be considered to have emotional and behavioral disorders as their most obvious problem (the ED category in the federal law). As we discuss later, the ED special education category under federal law overlaps with the group of children and youth known to have a variety of mental health difficulties. The kids typically have similar difficulties regardless of what they're called.

We could consider children with a wide variety of labels and conditions. For example, we could discuss those who are said to have a developmental disability or those with intellectual disabilities (formerly called mental retardation). Lots of kids with special needs are neglected, and their neglect is outrageous. As we said, though, our major focus is on those who have mental health problems.

Most children with seriously impairing emotional or behavioral problems—no, not those just having a little trouble, but those with problems that mental health experts judge to be *really* bad—get *no treatment at all*. Nothing. They don't get special education, and they don't get any other treatment for mental health problems, such as counseling or psychotherapy or medical prescriptions. Even the few who do get special education or other treatment usually get help only after their need is so long-standing, so outrageous, so undeniable, so obvious, or so in-your-face that people can't stand it anymore. Often, any help children with even these obvious problems get is too little and too late. What they usually get is inadequate, ineffective intervention long after their problems first became clear. Their problems are allowed to grow so severe, so bad that their effective treatment is very, very difficult.

Most people understand that the longer you let a physical problem go before treating it, the harder it is to treat. We know that a physician's chances of treating an illness successfully go way down when something like cancer is in an advanced stage. But, for some reason, many people don't seem to understand that the same is true for mental health problems. They seem to expect miracles, to expect great outcomes regardless of the stage to which the emotional or behavioral problem has been allowed to progress.

> Most people understand that the longer you let a physical problem go before treating it, the harder it is to treat. But, for some reason, many people don't seem to understand that the same is true for mental health problems.

We should recognize the fact that children's difficult behavior is often the beginning stage of mental health problems that will, potentially, dog them all their lives. Most mental illness doesn't just appear suddenly in a normal person. Usually, its onset is insidious—subtle, difficult to tell from what's considered normal. And, with a few extraordinary exceptions like schizophrenia, the beginning stages—the *onset*—are *typically* first observed during childhood, sometimes even *early* childhood, or *early* adolescence. If we really want to prevent long-term problems, not to mention shorter-term but serious difficulties, then we have to get after these things before they get so bad, nip them in the bud, be more willing to step in early. But this is a topic we've written about a lot in professional journals and books, and it's the topic of our Chapter 5.

Classroom teachers should be among the first responders to these problems because these children's difficulties are typically most obvious in school. Just consider that children spend a lot of their time in school. And teachers have a basis for comparison. They're especially likely to observe that a child is an outlier, way different, not like typically developing children.

So, sad but true, most children with serious emotional or behavioral problems, including those with serious mental illness, are never identified for special education or any other form of mental health service (in a later chapter, we describe how special education can be a mental health service). But that doesn't mean they shouldn't be. It just means that's the way it is now. Many decades of research in special education and mental health consistently tell us that at least 5 percent of children have some type of serious, debilitating emotional or behavioral problem, yet less than 1 percent of children get special education or other mental health services.[8] Most of those with mental health problems are in regular classrooms with regular teachers, which is all the more reason we should look at regular classroom teachers as first responders.

It's totally unrealistic to assume that we can somehow increase by a factor of 5 the percentage of the child population getting special education and mental health services for emotional or behavioral problems. But it *is* realistic to expect that these children's difficulties will be recognized in school for what they are; that special education and related services for them will not be cut; that such services will be available to more of them; and that regular classroom teachers will be taught how to recognize and provide better education for them, though many such children will need special education.

Most adults don't understand these issues. They think that most children who really need special attention or other treatment for their mental health problems are identified and get such treatment. They know some children are uninsured against physical disease, but they don't realize that the problem is much, much worse when it comes to emotional or behavioral difficulties, including clear cases of mental illness. And they don't understand that neglecting these children's problems often leads not only to more serious difficulties but to lifelong dysfunction as well. The problems of these children often lead to incarceration, unemployment, family disruption, and reliance on what few services there are for adults who don't function well in everyday life. The neglect of problems that could be addressed early has a high price tag, both in human misery and in dollars. But we tend to be penny-wise and pound-foolish when it comes to services for children with

> But we tend to be penny-wise and pound-foolish when it comes to services for children with mental health problems, cutting budgets for the services they need without realizing that we're shooting ourselves in the fiscal foot.

mental health problems, cutting budgets for the services they need without realizing that we're shooting ourselves in the fiscal foot.[9] We don't see the real cost of neglect right away. We often don't see it until years later. But many people aren't concerned about future costs, only present costs. Cut taxes and budgets now, worry about the consequences later.

As we've suggested, most of the emotional and behavioral problems of children can be seen clearly by teachers. Schools must become the first responders to such problems. That is, like the fire-rescue squads that we now expect to respond to accidents and calls of distress, school personnel must respond to the problems they see brewing. Yes, we'd rather the "accidents" and other emergencies didn't happen in the first place, but when they do happen we need people who are, as the old expression has it, "Johnny-on-the-spot." But, teachers' appeals for help for students who have emotional or behavioral problems—incipient or raging mental health problems—are now often interpreted as overreactions, a reflection of teachers' desire for easier jobs, teachers' cultural insensitivity, or their "bleeding heart" liberalism, or something else. A dismissive or derogatory spin is put on their expressions of concern.

> But, teachers' appeals for help for students who have emotional or behavioral problems—incipient or raging mental health problems—are now often interpreted as overreactions, a reflection of teachers' desire for easier jobs, teachers' cultural insensitivity, or their "bleeding heart" liberalism, or something else.

The reality of our neglect of children with emotional or behavioral problems is truly scandalous, but this reality has been with us for years. Why do we let such scandalous neglect go on and on, year after year? The answers aren't obvious. They aren't clear to the casual observer. They aren't simple. And they're often hidden by good intentions or well-meaning actions with horrible but mostly predictable negative consequences. In subsequent chapters, we'll look at some of the reasons behind this scandal and some of the arguments that people use to justify it. We know it's a long-standing problem that's often carefully hidden from the public, sometimes with good intentions. It's a problem that will persist until the general public not only sees it clearly but finds it intolerable.

The Number of Children With Mental Health Problems

The best studies we have suggest that *at least* 5 percent of the child population needs mental health services for problems that significantly affect their ability to function in everyday life. This isn't counting those with some sort of autism (known as autism spectrum disorder, ASD) or those with intellectual disabilities (ID). If the population of the United States that's under 18 years of age is, say, 100 million, that would be about 5 million children who have serious mental health needs. That's a lot of children. Even if the population is only 50 million, 2.5 million are probably going to have serious mental health problems. That's still a lot of children. Do the math for the actual population of the United States, and you'll see how many kids we should be talking about. The population of the U.S. that is 18 and under is about 75 million, so if we use 5 percent, that would mean 3.75 million would be needing help for very serious mental health problems. However, fewer than a million students are identified for special education in the emotional disturbance, or ED, category. And, as we shall see, special education is the only mental health service most students with mental health problems receive.

Why is such a low percentage of youngsters with serious problems identified for special education because of their emotional and behavioral problems? We discuss that in more detail later when we address the small number of kids getting services. Suffice it to say here that the reasons are many and complex. Among the reasons are cost, fear of labeling and stigma, lack of services, and hostility toward students who are themselves hostile or cause problems.

One common question is: Are these disorders increasing? That's a difficult question to answer definitively in the case of mental health disorders not associated with autism or intellectual disability. This is because "emotional disturbance" and "mental health problems" are less clearly defined than are some other disabilities and developmental problems. Such disorders don't appear to be increasing, but the truth is that we really don't know. However, an increase in number or percentage of the population is not really the issue here. Even if there is no increase at all, it's clear that most of the kids with really serious, protracted emotional or behavioral problems aren't getting what they need—nowhere close.

We know that problems of various kinds can increase dramatically and that autism spectrum disorder (ASD) is an example. ASD is now diagnosed far more frequently than it was a decade or longer ago. ASD can range from relatively mild impairment, sometimes called Asperger's syndrome, to severe cases involving absence of speech and other problems. But, again, ASD is not the primary issue here. Mental health problems are. True, the neglect of children and adults with ASD is outrageous, too. That neglect can't be justified either. ASD is now a separate category for special education purposes under federal law, but it is also a disorder included in the DSM, the *Diagnostic and Statistical Manual* of the American Psychiatric Association. But children with mental health problems far outnumber those with ASD, and the neglect of those children is also a national disgrace.

We know that almost all children have behavior problems of some kind or other at some time in their lives. The vast majority of these children are normal. It's just normal to have some problems. Nearly everybody, including nearly every child, has a "quirk." But we're *not* talking about normal children, who are the vast majority. We're *not* talking about half or a quarter of the child population. We know that about one in five (about 20 percent) of children at some time have some type of problem serious enough that it could be diagnosed as a mental illness. But most of the problems these children have are short-lived. *We're not talking about them, either.* No, we're *not* talking about the children who have *serious but temporary* problems. We're talking about the roughly one in 20 children (about 5 percent; that would be at least one student in most classrooms in the U.S.) who have *serious, protracted problems that impair their functioning in everyday life and create serious distress or danger to themselves or others.* Their problems aren't just serious. They're long-term and likely to be lifelong if the children don't get early, effective help.

We could think about millions of children, but let's think about the percentage of the population involved. Probably, it's just as easy to think of 10 percent or 5 percent or 1 percent of the population as to think of 10 million or 5 million or 1 million children. Besides, as the population increases, the number of children we might talk about changes, whereas the percentage is likely to remain roughly the same. So, for purposes of our discussion, we'll talk about percentages, and if you want to translate those into numbers of children then you can multiply the population by the percentages to get them. Percentages can change, too, but that's another matter, and for starters it's enough to consider the percentages that research of the past 50 years or so has given us.

The 5 percent estimate of those who have serious mental health needs wasn't just pulled out of a hat. It's based on a consensus of many studies done over decades using a variety of criteria and research methods. In 2000, the U.S. Surgeon General, then Dr. David Satcher, issued a report from the Department of Health and Human Services. The report concluded, based on the accumulation of research data over a period of decades, that at least 5 percent of our population of children and youth have serious and protracted mental health needs. Many other studies and reports, including a 2013 report of the Centers for Disease Control and Prevention, have concluded that the 5 percent estimate is conservative, not a stretch, not an overblown figure, and that few of the children who need mental health services get them. You could also explore the 2016 report of Mental Health America.[10]

We could look at an old study of school children by special educators at the University of Minnesota, Rosalyn Rubin and Bruce Balow, in 1978 as an example.[11] They found, using a survey of teachers, that 7.4 percent of the child population were said by their teachers consistently, over a three-year time span, to have behavior problems. These weren't children who were said by just one teacher or two but by every teacher they had in three years to have behavior problems. Compared to other students, they had lower achievement test scores in language, reading, spelling, and arithmetic. They also had lower IQ scores than most children. They were significantly lower in socioeconomic status, significantly higher in grade retentions, and required more special services such as remedial reading, speech therapy, psychological evaluations, and so on. Supposing that a third of these children didn't really have serious, protracted mental health needs, you still end up with about 5 percent of the school population.

Even so, when it comes to the individual case, it's hard to know for sure who we're talking about. The following case is quite typical of the problems we'll be talking about. Does J. K. need mental health services, or is he one of those children who has some trouble but will be okay without being identified as needing treatment? Are the signs of impending trouble clear? Do we know enough in this case to make a call—*yes*, treat it or *no*, leave it alone? Experts might disagree about what to do. What do *you* think?

J. K.

J. K. is a fifth-grader with an IQ of 115. He doesn't have any significant physical anomalies or any significant delay in developing motor or language skills. He didn't have any particular academic difficulties until fourth grade. His academic performance was about average until last year, when his grades suddenly began to go bad. This year he's gotten mostly Ds and Fs.

J. K. wasn't known as a problem child in school until last year. But every teacher who has dealt with him in the past 18 months has commented on his frequent misbehavior. He's difficult to manage because of his frequently getting out of his seat, talking out, teasing, and having tantrums. He often defies his teachers and gets into arguments with his peers. His teachers see these problems as increasing. His belligerence recently resulted in several fights in and around school, including a fight in which another child was injured and required medical attention. Two weeks ago, he was caught shoplifting a bag of candy from the local drugstore. His teachers rate him as showing behavior problems more often than 90 percent of his schoolmates.

J. K. doesn't have any close friends, but sometimes he's tolerated by other boys who have similar behavior problems. He and his two older brothers live with his mother and stepfather, who don't give him much supervision. His parents have never shown much concern about his lack of school progress, and they've refused to recognize that anything, including his fights and shoplifting, is a significant problem.

J. K.'s teachers are very concerned about him for several reasons. He doesn't complete most of his academic work, and he's failing most subjects. He disrupts the class frequently by hitting or taunting other students or mumbling complaints about the teacher and assignments. He spends a lot of his time in class drawing tattoos on his arms with felt-tip pens. None of his three experienced teachers, who manage 63 fifth-graders as a team, has been able to establish a close relationship with him or produce significant improvement in his behavior.

Remember this case, because it illustrates a lot about the difficulty of knowing just where to make the cut, where to draw the line, whom to include and whom not to include among those needing mental health services. Just where to draw the line is *always* an issue, just because of the way the world is, because the criterion or criteria for *any* special program is a matter related to statistics.[12]

We can look at more recent studies of the need for mental health services, too. Remember the 2000 report of the Surgeon General on children's mental health? Here's an excerpt from the first paragraph of the summary of the conference on which that report was based:

> Many children have mental health problems that interfere with normal development and functioning. In the United States, one in ten children and adolescents suffer from mental illness severe enough to cause some level of impairment (Burns et al., 1995; Shaffer et al., 1996).... Recent evidence compiled by the World Health Organization indicates that by the year 2020, childhood neuropsychiatric disorders will rise proportionately by over 50 percent, internationally, to become one of the five most common causes of morbidity, mortality, and disability among children.[13]

Well, okay, the report says one in 10, and the actual need may really involve 10 percent of children. But let's assume that only half of those who have "some impairment" have really *serious and protracted* problems. So, one in 20 (5 percent) is certainly a relatively conservative guess based on this report. If you look at other large-scale studies of prevalence published even more recently, you'll see that a lot of adults with diagnoses like anxiety disorders and impulse control disorders reported that their problems started when they were children.[14]

The data are clear and overwhelming: Although a huge percentage of children have passing problems and a large percentage of children and adults could be diagnosed at some time in their lives as having a psychiatric disorder, a substantial percentage of children and youth have more than passing or minor problems. The problems of about 5 percent of children are severe and chronic, putting them clearly in the category of those who need treatment. That is, we have good reason to believe that the emotional or behavioral problems of at least 5 percent of children and youth are serious and protracted enough that there is no legitimate question about their need for mental health services. They obviously need effective treatment. The next question is: Do they get it?

The Small Percentage Getting Treatment

On the question of what portion of that 5 percent needing mental health services actually get help, the data are also pretty clear. The Surgeon General's report of 2000 included this statement:

> Yet, in any given year, it is estimated that about one in five of such children [i.e., those with serious, protracted, often disabling mental health problems] receive ... mental health services (Burns et al., 1995). Unmet need for services remains as high now as it was 20 years ago.[15]

We can conclude not only from this statement but also from various other government reports and research by professionals and advocacy organizations that about one-fifth of the children who need mental health services for serious, protracted problems actually get services. This is scandalous neglect, but it's not new.

You might be tempted to think that although only about one child in five with very substantial mental health needs gets what's typically thought of as mental health services, such as therapies available through mental hospitals or community mental health centers, things like special education take up the slack. Think again. Data from the U.S. Department of Education and the National Research Council show that less than 1 percent of the school population receives special education under the "emotionally disturbed" category, and researchers have found that most of the services provided for the small percentage who get any mental health services at all get most or all of their services through the

> You might be tempted to think that although only about one child in five with very substantial mental health needs gets what's typically thought of as mental health services, such as therapies available through mental hospitals or community mental health centers, things like special education take up the slack. Think again.

schools.[16] Even if you throw in half of those children identified as having learning disabilities, assuming that the children have been mislabeled, you don't get to 5 percent of the child population.

Any way you cut it, regardless of how you define children's mental health services, the mental health needs of children and youth in America are severely, one might even say grotesquely, neglected. Most kids with serious mental health problems get no treatment of any kind. Those who do get something often get long-delayed and inadequate intervention. Most don't get even a Band-Aid when they need much more. The Band-Aids don't do much good, feeding the misleading argument that treatment doesn't work anyway. The scandal of unmet needs is clear. Possible solutions to the problem are not. Occasionally, a very high-profile case in which the inadequacy of mental health services is obvious makes the news.[17] Sometimes, these cases involve children, but more often they involve adults.

As one U.S. senator put it, in spite of some increases in mental health care, "we are still nowhere near where we need to be in making sure that people who need treatment for mental illness and addiction can always get it." And one key strategy for getting closer to meeting the need, this senator found by consulting the National Alliance on Mental Illness, is working with schools and teachers.[18]

Of course, the Surgeon General's report of 2000 and the 2013 report of the Centers for Disease Control and Prevention aren't the only reports of the problem of neglecting children's mental health needs. You could go way, way back in the history of special education and mental health and find the same kind of problem.[19] Nothing much has changed regarding the small percentage of children receiving mental health services or the reasons such a large percentage get none since a meeting of experts resulted in the following conclusions, published by the National Mental Health Association (NMHA) in 1986.[20] The experts working with the NMHA concluded that a majority of children with serious mental health needs are never identified as such and consequently don't receive the services they require. The reasons are many, and they include at least the following:

◆ People are concerned about the stigma a child might experience from labeling.
◆ The definitions of "emotional disturbance," "behavioral disorder," and other terms and the criteria for eligibility for services are vague and vary among states.

◆ Identification procedures among states and localities lack consistency.

◆ States and localities may set limits on the number of children they will identify because of costs.

◆ A child may not be identified because few services or only inappropriate services are available in the community.

◆ The community may lack confidence in its ability to develop appropriate services because of a lack of funding or because the problems are difficult to serve.

◆ Lack of clarity among mental health clinicians on definitions and diagnoses compounds the difficulty of deciding that a child needs mental health services.

◆ Federal special education law explicitly excludes children who are "socially maladjusted," but the distinctions between social maladjustment and emotional disturbance are confusing and meaningless. This confusion in labeling can result in some children not being identified or served.

◆ Adults tend to identify children whose inappropriate behavior stands out as in-your-face misconduct and tend to overlook those who don't act out. In some communities, this results in disproportionate representation of black males and under-identification of females of all races, who may not be labeled as troublesome but have very serious mental health problems.

◆ Children with mental health needs tend to have more severe disabilities, compared to other disability categories, before they're identified; their problems are often ignored for a long time.

In addition, the problem of identifying and serving children with mental health needs is made worse by the hostile attitude of many people toward them—particularly the assumption that these children *could* control their misbehavior if they wanted to, that they are just being bad by choice. Yes, we'd like to believe that these circumstances have all changed for the better in the last quarter-century. The fact is, they haven't. If anything, they've gotten worse.

We'll consider in more detail in subsequent chapters these and other reasons for our society's failure to meet the mental health needs of children. But to those of us who have studied these problems over a period of decades, this is "same-old-same-old." In fact, as the unmet need for mental health services for children and youth has stayed the same or grown since the 1980s, American society's response has been to trim funding for social programs for those in need of mental health interventions, saving tax dollars—saving money *now* on early identification and treatment but costing lots more money *later* for a variety of services for social dysfunction. This is not smart thinking about money.

The neglect of mental health needs at all ages continues. But it's especially galling when it's children's needs that are neglected, especially *young* children's needs, especially needs that turn into long-term disasters. Professor Glen Dunlap and his colleagues who work with preschoolers and those in the primary grades summarized consensus statements regarding young children with behavior problems. One of their findings was that such children are too seldom identified and appropriate services for them are too often not provided.[21]

This is scandalous, indeed, but not a new story for those who know the facts and figures on mental health services for children. The bad news continues for children and youth of all ages. Researcher Jane Costello and her co-workers found that only a small percentage of children with serious psychiatric disorders receive treatment. They remarked that when the usual treatments for child and adolescent psychiatric disorders were ineffective, then lack of treatment might have been said to be merely regrettable. However, with today's better treatment options, this lack of identification and service is a major public health issue. Moreover, the tragedy of lack of mental health services is compounded by convincing evidence that most psychiatric disorders start early in children's lives, and the risk of disorders that begin in adulthood is often increased by childhood adversities. Disorders starting in the early years often come back again in adulthood. So, the public health problem is very clear, as is the importance of early intervention. However, the reality is quite different.[22]

We hope you're getting the picture that not only do most children with mental health needs, regardless of their age, get nothing—ever—but that we probably can recognize the signs early on that a child is headed for serious mental health trouble. What people usually do when they see problem behavior is nothing, or nothing much. They typically let things go until the problem is outrageous, or somebody gets hurt, or things get so bad that people are desperate for help, or the child ends up in jail.[23] Reconsider the case of J. K. that we presented earlier. If you think J. K. did not have serious problems that should be addressed by special education or other mental health services, what would it take—what additional information would you need—for you to decide that he should get it?

We know that most of the students who are eventually identified as needing special education for emotional or behavioral disorders have been known to have problems for *several years*, not months.[24] Dr. Philip Wang and his coauthors writing in the *Archives of General Psychiatry* in 2005 noted that many people with severe and impairing mental health problems reported long delays in their mental health treatment.[25] Furthermore, Dr. Wang and his colleagues noted, it's not just the severe problems of adults we should worry about but the lower-level problems that are left to fester and, eventually, trigger more severe disorders. And a lot of these problems start during the school years. Some studies indicate that neurological problems can cause psychiatric disorders that, if untreated, become more frequent, severe, spontaneous, and resistant to treatment. Furthermore, we have good reason to believe, based on careful studies of epidemiology, that school failure, teenage parenthood, unstable employment, early marriage, marital violence, and marital instability are all associated with the mental disorders that begin early in life and go untreated.

> Furthermore, we have good reason to believe, based on careful studies of epidemiology, that school failure, teenage parenthood, unstable employment, early marriage, marital violence, and marital instability are all associated with the mental disorders that begin early in life and go untreated.

Dr. Wang and colleagues went on to explain that individuals having one problem often developed one or more additional problems (comorbidity is the technical term). Lots of children in that 5 percent who have serious mental health needs have multiple problems. They're at risk for very bad problems that are likely to be long-term, even lifelong. A lot of the youngsters we're considering start having more and more problems as they get older. They're often headed for a lifetime of trouble, something that is very likely not only to cost them and others a lot of heartaches but eventually cost taxpayers a huge bundle more than effective early intervention would have cost.

Blaming Children, Parents, and Teachers

When children misbehave seriously or have some sort of mental health problem, our first tendency is to try to find someone to blame. Kids themselves, their parents, and their teachers are the easiest first targets. There's plenty of blame to go around, so they're all likely to come in for some shaming.

Our first tendency is to blame children themselves—to conclude that they are having problems of their own making. And there is just enough truth in that to encourage the thought that punishment will solve the problem. It certainly seems to make sense, looking at things from the usual adult's perspective, that kids should "lie in the beds they've made for themselves." But we'll see later how the tendency to blame kids for their own problems and punish the behavior we don't want to see is typically not effective.

Next up for blame are parents. If a child has an emotional or behavioral problem, it's tempting to say the parents are to blame for failing to offer appropriate nurturing or support, or for mismanaging the child's discipline. As one student studying the emotional and behavioral problems of children and youth put it, "Show me an emotionally disturbed child, and I'll show you an emotionally disturbed parent." Parents of children with severe problems know this kind of blaming well, even if they have other children without significant problems. Sometimes, parents of very difficult children respond with understandable frustration, and some parents do things that are unwise. But that doesn't mean they deserve the blame for the problems their kids are having. Nevertheless, there is such a thing as poor parenting, and there is just enough truth in the idea that parents can edge their children toward deviant behavior to justify automatic blame in the minds of some people.

Then, if we can't blame someone else for a child's problems at school—maybe even if we can—we tend to blame his or her teacher(s). After all, teachers have a lot of responsibility for children's development and are responsible for managing children during many or most of their waking hours during school days. In America, teachers are often considered to be "not the sharpest knives in the drawer," to be biased, and to be poorly trained. Again, this is sometimes true, and it's just enough truth to give many critics the ammunition they need to hurl unwarranted generalizations at teachers in general for being incompetent or worse. Asking teachers to deal with problems for which they have no training or inadequate training is abusive, and such abuse of teachers is abetted by the full inclusion movement that places students with emotional and behavioral disorders in regular classes, regardless of the nature or severity of the child's emotional or behavioral disability.[26]

Finding someone to blame for a child's mental health problem isn't very helpful. The cause of the problem usually isn't clear, and it's very seldom a single person or thing.

The Disproportionality and Over-Identification Issues

A common complaint is that children in some groups—males, African Americans, those of lower socioeconomic status, for example—are disproportionately identified for special education or other mental health services. Such observations were included in the 1986 report of the National Mental Health Association (previously mentioned; see note 17). We note that such disproportional identification—particularly the presumed over-identification of African American children based on comparison of their percentage of the child population and their percentage of children identified for special education—has been very controversial for a very long time.

The disproportionality issue is, indeed, like "quicksand," in that the definitions of emotional disturbance used in many state laws and federal law and regulations are ambiguous, confusing, and in some cases unintelligible.[27] This fact allows charges of racism or racial bias and denial regardless of what one concludes about the causes or meaning of disproportionality. It encourages suspension of judgment, such that the least damaging statements reflect a firm agnosticism and calls for additional research.[28] Nevertheless, behavior that is clearly antisocial, reflects denial of reality, or demonstrates extreme social withdrawal has been recognized as deviant in many different cultures and throughout history.[29] We are not discussing here those children whose behavior is marginal, only a little problematic, or only situational and temporary. Rather, we are concerned with those who are having severe, long-standing problems, whose deviation from the "normal" or "acceptable" should be recognized today in any group as having very serious problems. Moreover, research suggests that the same basic principles of instruction in academics and management of behavior apply to children regardless of their ethnicity, gender, or religion.[30]

Suffice it to say here, the notion that mental health problems are *often* mistaken and that *many* of the students identified are merely "culturally different" and do not actually have emotional or behavioral disorders has been thoroughly debunked.[31] In fact, research is now showing that African-American students who need services for mental health problems or other school problems are, if anything, *under*-identified compared to Caucasian students who are similar in achievement and behavior.[32] Part of the scandal of neglect of children's mental health needs might be attributed to the mistaken belief that certain groups of students have been over-identified. The data simply do not support the myth of over-identification. We conclude that the neglect of minority students' mental health and their exclusion from special education for children with emotional and behavioral disorders fits the shameful pattern of neglect of these children's other needs.

> The notion that mental health problems are often mistaken and that many of the students identified are merely "culturally different" and do not actually have emotional or behavioral disorders has been thoroughly debunked.

A Place to Start

We need a systematic analysis of the problem, the scandal. And that implies some sort of starting place, to make sure we know what we're talking about. If we want to address this scandal effectively, then we have to start with some basics.

We think starting with the measurement of mental health makes the most sense. How do we know? How do we judge? What makes us believe that children have mental health problems anyway? This is basically a measurement issue, so we consider measurement in the next chapter.

Notes

1. Earley (2006), Powers (2017), Warner (2010).
2. E.g., Achenbach and Nutt (2016), Dionne (2016), Fisher (2016), Kagan (2016); see also Kauffman and Badar (2017). Bullying threatens the mental health of many children (e.g., Harris, 2017)

and can reflect emotional/mental health issues of either the bully or the bullied or both.

3. See Abernathy (2017), Dionne, Mann, and Ornstein (2014), Lozada (2014). Children and adults can be both bad and "mad," as wretchedly bad behavior and mental illness overlap. As some point out, calling Donald Trump "mentally ill" is a serious disservice to many people with mental illness, few of which exhibit his level of narcissism (see Wilson & Frances, 2017). Regarding imitation, research on imitation strongly suggests that models who are powerful and said to have desirable characteristics are more likely to be imitated than are those lower in status (see Hallenbeck & Kauffman, 1995).

4. See Franken (2017, chapter 38).

5. Karp (2017).

6. We use the term or label EBD as a singular noun for the general category of problems that encompasses various subtypes or subcategories. However, we also recognize that EBD refers to a variety of disorders and therefore could be considered plural (although we do not use "EBDs" to indicate this). In short, our use of EBD may be considered singular or plural in a given sentence.

7. Mattison (2014) describes the importance of teachers' understanding of DSM categories, especially special education teachers' understanding of them.

8. For information about these estimates and services, see Costello, Egger, and Angold (2005), Donovan and Cross (2002), Forness, Freeman, Paparella, Kauffman, and Walker (2012), Kauffman and Landrum (2018b), Kauffman, Mock, and Simpson (2007), Kessler, Chiu, Demler, and Walters (2005), Lane, Menzies, Oakes, and Kalberg (2012), Mattison (2014); National Mental Health Association (1986), U.S. Department of Health and Human Services (2000), annual reports to Congress on implementation of the Individuals with Disabilities Act, and Wang, Berglund, Olfson, Pincus, Wells, and Kessler (2005).

9. See Kendziora (2004), especially pp. 341–342.

10. See Forness et al. (2012), Kauffman and Landrum (2018b), Kauffman, Mock, and Simpson (2007), Mattison (2014); see also Centers for Disease Control and Prevention (2013, May 17). Mental health surveillance among children—United States, 2005–2011 (Retrieved May 30, 2013 from www.cdc.gov/mmwr/preview/mmwrhtml/su6202a1.htm?s_cid=su6202a1_w); see also Mental Health America (2016, retrieved November 7, 2016 from www.mentalhealthamerica.

net/issues/2016-state-mental-health-america-youth-data. Useful information can also be found at the Children's Mental Health Network at www.cmhnetwork.org.

11. Rubin and Balow (1978).
12. Kauffman and Lloyd (2017), Mattison (2014). For additional case descriptions, see Kauffman and Landrum (2018a).
13. U.S. Department of Health and Human Services. (2000). *Report of the Surgeon General's conference on children's mental health: A national action agenda*. Washington, DC: Author.
14. See, for example, Kessler et al. (2005) and note studies reviewed by Warner (2010) and Powers (2017).
15. U.S. Department of Health and Human Services. (2000). *Report of the Surgeon General's conference on children's mental health: A national action agenda*. Washington, DC: Author.
16. Evans, Rybak, Strickland, and Owens (2014), Forness et al. (2012), Kauffman and Landrum (2018b).
17. See McCrummen (2014).
18. Franken (2017, pp. 310–311).
19. Kauffman and Landrum (2006).
20. National Mental Health Association (1986); see also Kauffman et al. (2008).
21. Dunlap et al. (2006).
22. Costello et al. (2005), Schaaff (2016).
23. Earley (2006), Warner (2010).
24. Duncan, Forness, and Hartsough (1995).
25. Wang et al. (2005, pp. 610–611).
26. Kauffman and Badar (2016), Kauffman, Felder, Ahrbeck, Badar, and Schneiders (in press), Kauffman, Lloyd, Baker, and Riedel (1995). For more information on inclusion, see Anastasiou, Gregory, and Kauffman, (in press); Kauffman, Anastasiou, Badar, and Hallenbeck (in press); Kauffman, Anastasiou, Badar, Travers, and Wiley (2016); Kauffman and Badar (2014); and Kauffman, Bantz, and McCullough (2002).
27. Sullivan (2017).
28. Carrero, Collins, and Lusk (2017).
29. see Kauffman and Landrum (2006, 2018b), Scull (2015).
30. Kauffman, Conroy, Gardner, and Oswald (2008); see also Anastasiou and Kauffman (2010, 2012).
31. Forness et al. (2012); Kauffman and Anastasiou (in press).
32. Anastasiou and Kauffman (2010), Anastasiou, Morgan, Farkas, and Wiley (2017), Kauffman and Anastasiou (in press).

2

Measurement of Mental Health

Our concern here is measurement of mental health and mental illness. At first, our discussion might seem to be a digression. But an important point here is that measurement of mental health is, in many ways, like the measurement of anything else. That is, measurement of *anything* involves some core ideas and principles, and the measurement of mental health becomes less mysterious if we understand some of the basic principles of measurement *per se*.

We might start by remembering that when we really care about something, we find some way to measure it, even if measuring it means only "keeping track" of it or making a quick, informal judgment or assigning it to a category. So, we might conclude that if we really care about mental health, we'll find a way of measuring it.

Consider measurement of some other things. We care about how our children grow, so we measure and keep track of their height and weight. Pediatricians do this, and many parents do it themselves. Time and distance are important in sports, so officials keep careful track of them and make careful judgments about them. Sports fans care about statistics related to teams and players because these measures reveal how well a team or athlete is doing compared to others. We measure things like body temperature, blood pressure, heart rate, and so on because of what these measurements tell us and because we want medicine based on science. We even ask people to rate their pain on a scale from 1 to 10 so we can measure something intangible. These measurements and others give us important information about physical health or illness and whether it's getting better or worse. And we know that we can't investigate something scientifically if it can't be measured somehow.[1] In a world without measurement, we can't make good judgments, and accountability is not possible in the absence of measurement, even if the measurement is somebody's judgment (simply because they have to say what criteria they're using and how). The same is true when it comes to mental health.

Some things are far easier to measure than others. Height and weight are a lot easier to measure than intelligence or mental health. The units we use to measure some things seem natural or obvious to us in contemporary life, and some measurements are more familiar to us than others. Feet and inches, pounds and ounces, miles, kilometers, even IQ and light years don't seem unfamiliar, but things like percentiles and standard deviations on various tests might throw us because they're relatively unfamiliar. Furthermore, although measures of distance between points are familiar to nearly everyone, measures of social deviance are not. People often don't know what to make of measures of social deviance. Some measurements require explanation if people are going to understand them. Measurement of mental health is often one of those things.

Mental Health and Its Measurement

We need some sort of measure of children's mental health because we care about it and want to know whether a given measurement means they need treatment. We also need measurement to help us judge whether a child's mental health is getting better or getting worse. But we also must recognize that mental health is a relatively difficult thing to measure and that many of the measures and units used to measure mental health require explanation. That's in part because we're measuring something intangible, in this case people's judgment of their internal states or behavior, or the conduct of someone else. And there is inevitably a subjective element in doing this. But, measure we must, unless we don't care about mental health or don't care whether our judgments are based to the maximum extent on scientific evidence. And we try to make the measurement as objective as we can, knowing objectivity is never total.

Accuracy of Measurement

Some measures are more accurate than others, but no measure is absolute—so perfect that there is no possibility of error. We have to recognize the limitations of our measurement of anything. All measurement is less than infinitely precise, and we need to understand the level of precision and error that applies to our measurements. And in measuring mental health, we're going to find considerable error regardless of how careful and precise we try to be.

All measures of mental health and mental illness are very controversial. That is, none of the ways mental health is measured will be universally accepted or thought by everyone to be valid—an *absolutely real and precise* measure of a person's mental health. Probably it's important to realize that this is true of nearly everything we measure in the psychology of human beings—things like intelligence, academic knowledge, perceptions, biases, and any other aspect of a person's mental life. Somebody, often someone with considerable influence, will contend that the measure, the scale, the test, or judgment by whatever standard is used is flawed, unreliable, or biased.

As we've said, the fact is that no measurement is perfect, especially mental measurements. Measures of time and distance (including height and length and weight) are pretty well accepted as valid and reliable, even though they always entail some level of error or inaccuracy, simply because no measurement is absolute. We might get really close to infinite precision in the measurement of some things in the material world, like speed or weight or measurements required for making tools or machinery. However, we know there's going to be more error in mental measurement than in measurement of material things. Mental measurements (that is, measurement of anything psychological) are particularly vulnerable to criticism for being wrong or inaccurate or invalid or unreliable. They always have a certain amount of error, but they're not always way off or invalid.

Effects and Noneffects of Measurement

A very silly objection to mental measurements is that you can't measure anything without changing it (the Heisenberg principle of uncertainty is sometimes invoked in making this assertion). But that principle of uncertainty (Heisenberg's) applies *only* to measurements of subatomic particles, and even then to vanishingly small measurements. Heisenberg's uncertainty principle has no application at all to things we can see with the naked eye, and its extension to mental measurements is pure poppycock. So, don't be fooled by high-sounding discussions of Heisenberg's principle as if it means anything for measurement of things other than subatomic particles.[2]

The act of measuring mental health usually has very few, if any, effects on what is being measured. However, *what people do with a measurement they obtain may well have effects on mental health.* Measurement may be used in a variety of ways, and it may be appropriate or inappropriate, helpful or unhelpful. Any measurement may be used to demean someone, to make invidious comparisons, or in some unjustified way to do harm. However, measurement may also be used to help someone understand just how an individual is different from most, what is needed, or what progress is being made in treatment. It's very important to use measurement in ways that enhance understanding and treatment. We must be careful not to abuse measurement and to understand that *the abuse of measurement doesn't mean measurement is the problem.* People may abuse anything that can be used well by others, so we must be determined to see that measurement *itself* is not the problem.

General Principles of Measurement

Let's start with what we know about all measurements of things we can see with the unaided eye. Take height, for example. Consider some of the things we know about measuring height, whether it's the height of people or of buildings. We'll start with these more objective things because they'll help us understand the measurement of more subjective things like aggressiveness.

First, there's the scale of measurement. We could measure height to the nearest inch or half-inch or quarter-inch or eighth-inch, or an even smaller unit. Likewise, in measuring some aspect of mental health we might, for example, count the number of hits someone else (or engages in another aggressive act) per day, per hour, per minute, and so on.

Second, if we decide on a scale (i.e., how fine or accurate we want to be), then we could decide that there are tall people and short people. But, what is the meaning of "tall" or "short"? Obviously, we could draw the line for either wherever we think we're justified in doing so. Is 5 feet 6 inches short for a man, or should it be 5 feet 5 inches? Or something else, like 5 feet 5.5 inches? Are only those men and women who are 6 feet 6.25 inches or taller to be considered "tall"? Should the same designations of tallness and shortness apply to both men and women? At what chronological age does the designation apply? You may have your own opinion. Someone else may disagree with you. Obviously, any choice of a "cut point" for tall or short is just an arbitrary decision—one that could be changed by a quarter of an inch (or whatever scale or level of precision might be). And whatever the choice of a cut point for defining tall or short, some people will miss it narrowly, just by a little.

Suppose we didn't have cut points at all? Then we'd have a more subjective judgment of short and tall. Perhaps you see how the problem is related to measuring mental health. At what point do we say that a child is too aggressive or is depressed or has an obsessive-compulsive disorder? Just how different does the child have to be from most kids to be said to have a mental health problem of any kind? Where do we draw the line, who does it, and what are their criteria?

Some people will argue that we should just avoid measuring and comparing kids. But that line of argument just avoids several realities. It avoids the reality that if we care about something, we measure it in every way we can. It also avoids the reality that measurement requires or at least inevitably results in comparisons. And it avoids the realities of the mathematical principles we call statistics.

People can ignore any realities they want or reduce them to trivialities. But ignoring realities doesn't destroy them. It just makes for the kind of poor thinking that we don't want children, much less adults, to use. For example, someone might assume that everyone can be at or above the average. Statistically—mathematically—this is just impossible. So, when somebody suggests that we should raise our standards and improve our schools so that *all* children will perform at a certain level, they're obviously talking about something that simply can't and won't ever happen, regardless how good our schools become—unless *all* doesn't really mean each and every one. *Don't get us wrong! We think schools can and should do a better job of teaching all children. But teaching better and ignoring statistical realities are two different things entirely.*

> When somebody suggests that we should raise our standards and improve our schools so that all children will perform at a certain level, they're obviously talking about something that simply can't and won't ever happen, regardless how good our schools become.

So, what does all this have to do with measuring mental health? A lot, actually. We need to understand that whenever we measure something, we're faced with the realities of statistics, which is to say mathematics. Some people may consider these realities "problems" or otherwise relegate them to avoidable "artifacts," but that's sort of like saying that sums or subtrahends are "problems" or "artifacts" of math.

One of the realities of measuring mental health is that regardless of how we go about measuring it, we'll get a statistical distribution of scores. That will be true every single time, no exceptions. That's just the way the math of statistics works. Therefore, we have to use what we know about statistics in thinking about mental health problems.[3]

Thinking More About Measurement of Mental Health Problems

In thinking about mental health, statistics are important. However, we're not going to focus on statistics. We're just going to think about measurement in a way that makes sense to us (and, we hope, to you), and in doing that we'll keep the matter of statistical terms and formulas for calculating things in the background, just as we have so far. But there are some additional things to think about regarding the measurement of mental health.

Before going any further, we have to think about how mental health or mental illness is currently being measured. That is, what methods or instruments (what tests, what scales or rankings or judgments) are used to decide that a child has mental health problems? How do people use these things to determine mental health or illness? We need to consider both the instruments (that is, questionnaires or rating scales or guidelines) and the statistical criteria for drawing a line or choosing a cut point for deciding that a child has a mental health problem.

There is no standardized test as such for mental health. That is, we don't have a "mental health test" that's exactly like an intelligence test. So, we can't give a test that gives us something equivalent to an IQ. However, the same statistical principles apply to IQ and assessment of mental health. There are questionnaires or scales that parents or teachers might fill out about a child, and there are guidelines that psychiatrists and clinical psychologists use for judging a child's mental health. Usually, mental health professionals use the guidelines in the current edition of the American Psychiatric Association's *Diagnostic and Statistical Manual* or DSM.

Psychologists or educators might use rating scales that give them scores that they can compare to norms. A given rating scale might have many items—50, or even 100 or more. The items (descriptions or questions) might be things like *"Tattles on others," "Is shy," "Clings to parents," "Complains of loneliness," "Argues," "Doesn't obey," "Confused or seems to be in a fog," "Steals," "Dislikes school," "Cries a lot,"* and so on that describe problems. And for items like this a parent or teacher might give a rating ranging from, say, *1—never* to *5—very frequently*. However, some rating scales also include descriptions of behavioral strengths or competencies—things that describe the kind of behavior that's associated with robust mental health, like *"expresses emotions appropriately in difficult social situations."* Usually, the rating scale asks either a parent or a teacher to judge whether a described behavior or characteristic is seen *never, seldom, sometimes, often,* or *constantly.* Or the instrument might ask whether the item is *not at all like, somewhat or sometimes like,* or *very or often like* a child. So, essentially, the teacher or parent is asked to rate each item on a scale of, say, 1–3, 1–4, or 1–5, and the numbers are then totaled up to get a score.

Some instruments include self-ratings, peer ratings, or both. That is, the child is asked to rate his or her own behavior or classmates are asked to rate the child's behavior. Questions on self-reports might include things like *"My parents bug me a lot," "I often break my parents' rules,"* or *"I seem to get into a lot of fights."* Peer ratings also typically include items describing behavior. Self-reports can be very useful in judging not only what a child thinks about himself or herself but how his or her self-perceptions correspond to those of teachers, parents, or peers. Sometimes self-reports pick up problems that parents or teachers didn't know about. Also, the child may see himself or herself in positive terms that are very different from how parents, the teacher, or peers see things. The case of James illustrates how this might work out. In this case, ratings by teachers and classmates were used to assess the student's behavior. Notice how different James's perceptions of himself are from those of his teachers and classmates.

James

James's middle school teachers report that he has tantrums, uses obscene language, shows sad emotions, and is neglected by his peers. He was originally referred for possible eligibility for special education (the first step toward special education) when he was in the third grade. He was having difficulty in all academic areas and had poor interactions with his peers. He had more difficulty than most children working with others in a group. By the end of third grade, his acting-out behaviors were increasing. He was also teased by his classmates and showed symptoms of depression, such as almost total lack of interest in activities that previously were of interest to him. These problems continued through the fourth grade. His teachers reported that he made little progress in reading and writing. His teachers also observed that he was easily frustrated, quit without trying, and had developed obsessive-compulsive behaviors.

By the fifth grade, James still was reading at a pre-primer level. Behavior ratings showed that his self-concept was at or above average in spite of the low ratings of his behavior by his teachers and classmates. James described himself as well-liked, able to handle social situations successfully, a good student, and able to turn in work on time. His teachers countered with observations that his peers avoided him, he had low social skills, low academic competence, and required frequent reminders to complete his assignments.[4]

It's very common for people to believe that children with mental health problems always have a low self-concept, and many people in fact seem to believe that a low self-concept is typically the cause of emotional or behavioral problems. James's case shows that children with very serious problems may have unrealistically high self-concepts, too. But besides comparisons like those presented in James's case, it's important to consider the kinds of scores a rating scale might give us.

You might note also that James had serious academic and social problems years before his possible eligibility for special education was even considered. This is typical, unfortunately, and in Chapter 5 we discuss this problem of reluctance to deal with problems preventively.

That is, we give more attention to how failure to deal with problems early fosters the scandalous neglect of kids.

Behavior rating scales might have subscales, like *externalizing* (aggressive, acting-out behavior) and *internalizing* (withdrawn, depressed, immature, or otherwise internal troubles). On any given subscale or for the total score on a rating scale, the person using the instrument might be able to say that the child's score was as high or higher than, say 40 percent, 50 percent, 80 percent, or 95 percent of the "norm" or comparison group, which is usually an unselected, random group of kids or a group considered to be "normal." Sometimes, whoever designed and "normed" the instrument suggests a "clinical" range, meaning that a score falls into the range of scores of children who are receiving mental health services.

Sometimes ratings are supplemented by direct observation of behavior in typical social contexts. A trained observer, like a psychiatrist or psychologist or specially trained teacher, might watch the child in the classroom or on the playground or at home, for example, and keep track of how the child behaves. They look at what the child does and the circumstances surrounding the behavioral incidents. This is often very helpful in making judgments because it is based on more objective, observable behavior. But, of course, these observations, like behavioral ratings or any other kind of information, have to be interpreted—judged as to their meaning, compared to ratings or observations of typical children of the same age and gender. Observations are more valuable when they're longer and multiple observers see similar behavior and reach a consensus. Short observations of a single individual may be seriously misleading.

Sometimes, no actual rating scale or other pencil-and-paper instrument is used and no direct observations of the child's behavior in typical context is made. Rather, a psychologist or psychiatrist interviews the child (and perhaps parents or other adults who know the child well) and makes a judgment based on experience and the guidelines provided by a diagnostic and statistical manual.[5] This kind of judgment is sort of like the ratings of judges in an athletic contest. It's based on the judge's looking at a lot of cases and being trusted to make a good call based on his or her qualifications.

Sometimes all of these ways of measuring are used: rating scales, direct observations, and clinical interviews. These may involve the school, although sometimes they do not. Regardless, trust of a professional's clinical judgment of a child's mental health is based on the same kind of trust we place in referees or critics or professionals in other lines of work to make good calls. Can they be wrong? Surely, they can. But most of the time, unless they're really incompetent and ought to be removed, we go by their call because (1) they usually know what they're doing and (2) we've given them the authority or power to make the call.

What kinds of things does a psychologist or psychiatrist consider when making a judgment? Usually, he or she will consider (1) the particular difficulty the child has, (2) the circumstances of the child's life, (3) medical conditions that might contribute to an emotional or behavioral problem, and (4) how well the child is functioning in everyday life. The child's behavior isn't considered out of context or without attention to these other factors. In considering what diagnosis to make, the mental health professional will also use guidelines regarding the length of time the problem has existed and the number of symptoms or behaviors in a list that the child shows. For example, in diagnosing a "conduct disorder" (repeatedly, persistently violating the rights of others or age-appropriate expectations) the mental health professional making the judgment will consider how long and to what extent the child has shown aggression toward people or animals, property destruction, theft or deceit, and violation of rules established by parents or teachers. The person doing the diagnosis will likely consider not just ratings or behavioral observations or reports but all sources of information and how well they agree.

> Explicit in the statistical norms for any scale that might be used and implicit in any judgment call is this idea: *there is no set and clear standard or score that removes all judgment.*

Whether we rely on a score on some rating scale or instrument or whether we go by the call of a referee (in the case of mental health, usually a psychologist or psychiatrist trained to make such calls), statistics are involved. Explicit in the statistical norms for any scale that might be used and implicit in any judgment call is this idea: *there is no set and clear standard or score that removes all judgment.* The judgment might be right, or it might be wrong. If it's wrong, it could be wrong either way: the judgment could be that the child *has* a problem when he or she actually *doesn't*; or the judgment could be that the child *doesn't* have a problem when he or she actually *does*. Either mistake is bad, and nobody's judgment is *always* right, so we really have to think about which kind of mistake is worse and try to avoid it.[6]

In thinking about mental illness, including children's, we need to understand the tools used to measure and define it—both the ways the children's behavior is measured or evaluated and the statistical realities that are associated with measurement. We've already discussed the various measures—rating scales, direct observation, and interviews. So, it's really a matter of thinking about the statistical realities involved with all measurements. The truth is that we pick a point on a distribution and say that those on one side of it *are* mentally ill and those on the other side of it *are not* mentally ill. One unavoidable reality is that if we don't have such a line, then nobody gets identified as having crossed it. Another unavoidable reality is that the closer we move the line of demarcation to the average, the more cases of uncertainty we are going to encounter.[7] If we do have a line, then we always have people *close to it* or *on it* but not clearly over it. And if you think about it, you'll see that the closer the line is to the average, the more individuals we're talking about. Remember the case of James? Which side of the line is he on? Some people might judge that his problems aren't quite bad enough to be over the line and into mental illness; others might judge that he's clearly over the line.

But here's a problem we're faced with. What should we do when we're in doubt, as we are going to be in many cases? Should we run the risk of putting the child on the side of mental health or on the side of mental illness? When we're uncertain, if we think that identifying the child and making him or her eligible for treatment is likely to be more helpful than harmful, then we'll run the risk of putting the child on the side of mental illness. But if we think that identifying him or her and making the child eligible for treatment is likely to be more hurtful than helpful, then we'll run the risk of putting the child on the side of mental health. We think you can clearly bet on this—mental health professionals are very, very unlikely to put children on the side of mental illness for no good reason. Most mental health professionals see the value of treatment. That is, if the child is judged to have a serious mental health problem, then professionals believe that treatment is something to be wanted and embraced, not avoided and denigrated.

> We think you can clearly bet on this—mental health professionals are very, very unlikely to put children on the side of mental illness for no good reason.

Unfortunately, it appears that when it comes to this question of which side of the line is less risky, too many people go with the idea that it's better *not* to identify the child and make him or her eligible for special education or other mental health service.[8] Apparently, perhaps out of deference to parents or out of fear of court action or for ideological reasons, too many people conclude that special education is more bad than good, a raw deal. The assumption that special education or other mental health service is a bad deal is, itself, scandalous. The data don't suggest that it is and, in fact, suggest that the children who get early, effective special education are better off than those who don't.[9] But the larger scandal is that such a small percentage—perhaps 20 percent—of the children that mental health professionals routinely identify as having serious, protracted mental health needs get treatment of any kind. They don't get services even after the best measurement we have indicates that they need help.

Differences in Measurement and Services

It may have occurred to you that the percentage of the child population considered to have severe mental health problems (about 5 percent) is about five times higher than the percentage receiving any sort of mental health intervention. But the percentage receiving special education in the emotionally disturbed (ED) category is *even less than 1 percent* (more like .7 or .8 percent). This low percentage is especially discrepant from the 5 percent said to have severe mental health problems.

There is a potential explanation for the extraordinarily low percentage of children with mental health problems receiving special education. The potential explanation is related to the federal definition of ED.[10] The federal definition includes the phrase "which adversely affects educational performance." If "educational performance" is interpreted to mean only academic achievement, then a child who is testing at grade level is highly unlikely to be considered to have mental health problems under special education law and regulation. Yet, we know that some children with very significant mental health issues perform on grade level in school. So, the federal definition of ED needs to be changed to recognize the fact that children may have serious mental health issues, yet not have academic performance deficits that qualify them for special education under current law. We ought to interpret "educational performance" to mean more than academics.[11]

We also know that mental health problems are not confined to school and that we see them played out in a variety of circumstances. The kids we see demonstrating their mental health problems in the community are often having difficulties of various kinds in school, too. In fact, a good definition of mental health problems includes the requirement that the problem be exhibited in more than a single setting. Often, those with mental health problems are drawn to others who encourage deviant behavior and goad other members of the group toward more serious misconduct. Very often, such behavior is upsetting to others, though it is not illegal. Consider the experiences of a young female teacher who encountered such behavior of a group of youngsters at a mall:

The crowd at the mall was a surprise, but more disconcerting to both me and my three-year-old son was the noise level and the rowdiness, both of which were due to throngs of teens roaming the mall, many in groups of eight or 10 or more. They were laughing loudly and engaging in horseplay, but I was surprised at their roughness and rowdiness and use of bad language. They pushed and shoved each other, often into other shoppers. They made no attempt at all to conceal their frequent use of profanity and extremely coarse language, especially about members of the opposite sex. In fact, they were seeming to enjoy shocking others with their trash-talking. There were plenty of adults around, but everyone seemed to be ignoring these kids and their behavior. I guess they found it normal teenage conduct. Either that or, like me, they were bothered by it but didn't know what to do.

One group of kids had me quite unnerved, as they seemed to notice my son and me in particular; they gestured directly toward us at the food court, and seemed to be cracking jokes about the baby stroller or the stuffed animal my son held. I could not fully hear everything they said—except that the profanity was clear. What bothered me even more about this group in particular was their age. I estimated they were not more than 12 or 13 years old, and at least one in this group of four boys and two girls looked no older than 10.

Bothered by the crowd and the youngsters' behavior, I decided to cut the evening short and go back to the parking lot. As I did, one of the members of this group of six called to me— actually to my son. "Hey, little man, let me see your elephant." I can't describe my emotions at that moment, and in fact I'm not quite sure what I felt.

I know I was shocked that they were speaking to us, but I was also very angry. Probably, I was a little frightened, too. I thought

I might be in danger, that this might be something more than he, my three-year-old, being exposed to dreadful profanity and behavior I'd rather not have him see. I had just heard these six teens talking graphically about sexual encounters, tossing racial slurs (their group included African Americans, Caucasians, and one Asian teen), and homophobic taunts to each other and even to total strangers. And now they were talking to me and my three-year-old in a way I found threatening

My gut told me to ignore them, but as we had to pass right by them to get to the parking lot, I decided to let them know I didn't appreciate their behavior in front of my child. A confrontation was more than I wanted, however, so I put on my best teacher-face and merely gave the young man who had spoken the sternest look I could muster.

To my surprise and dismay, however, he looked me right in the eye and shot back almost immediately, "What the [expletive] are you looking at, [expletive]?" I'm sure they all saw the stunned look on my face, as I really didn't know what to do or say. Of course, I wanted to tear into this young man, asking who he thought he was to talk to me or my son or anyone that way. But I did my best to ignore his question, and wheeled right past them and out the door toward my car.

The kids all hooted as we passed them by. It was a long way across the dark parking lot to my car. I really wished I could spot the elderly security guard we had talked to earlier on our way into the mall.[12]

The behavior of the group of teens this woman encountered in the mall may be common, but it does not reflect good mental health. Too often in our society, behavior that is inappropriate and indicates mental health problems is shrugged off, seen as normal, simply because it is not unusual for some aspect of its context. True, sometimes people are put off by behavior or are afraid and don't know what to do.

A lot of our measurement of mental health and mental

> Too often in our society, behavior that is inappropriate and indicates mental health problems is shrugged off, seen as normal, simply because it is not unusual for some aspect of its context.

health problems starts out, at least, with gut reaction to behavior. We may see behavior at first glance—sometimes our only way of assessing it—as normal or deviant, inappropriate or unacceptable. Clearly, the young woman described above encountered behavior of kids in the mall that she considered inappropriate. Sometimes, we may have to be satisfied with general judgments, clearly a crude measurement of the problem. More sophisticated measurement is desirable, but sometimes not possible. Crude measurement—judgment that something is in bounds or out of bounds—is often important. The lines we draw for concluding that something is okay or not okay are important. Sometimes, we need to change kids' behavior. Sometimes, we don't need to change it but do need to change our level of tolerance.[13] Drawing the line is often a real challenge.

> The lines we draw for concluding that something is okay or not okay are important. Sometimes, we need to change kids' behavior. Sometimes, we don't need to change it but do need to change our level of tolerance.

Measurement of More Specific Problems

So, next we need to consider how measurement of mental health is related to more specific problems. We also need to think about how mental illness is related to special education for children and youth who fall into the federal category of ED. In the next chapter, we consider more specific kinds of problems kids have and how these problems are related to both mental health and special education. And although it's often very difficult, we must draw the lines at which mental health problems begin.

Notes

1. Kauffman (2011); see also Alexandrova (2017) and her comments on measurement of mental health and Lewis (2017) for his account of how psychologist Kahneman focused on measurement of psychological phenomena.
2. See Kauffman (2010) for further discussion.

3. These concepts are discussed further by Kauffman (2011) and Kauffman and Lloyd (2017); see also Imray and Colley (2017).

4. Rewritten from Lambros, Ward, Bocian, MacMillan, and Gresham (1998).

5. E.g., Shaffer et al. (1996); see also Lane et al. (2012).

6. Kauffman (2007), Lane et al. (2012).

7. See Kauffman and Lloyd (2017). For further discussion of uncertainties of judgments in a variety of circumstances, see Lewis (2017).

8. Kauffman (2007), Kauffman et al. (2007), Kauffman and Landrum (2018b).

9. See Kauffman (2008, 2010), Kauffman, Hallahan, Pullen, and Badar (2018), Mattison (2014).

10. Kauffman and Landrum (2018b).

11. Forness and Knitzer (1992).

12. Rewritten from Kauffman and Landrum (2018a).

13. Kauffman, Pullen, Mostert, and Trent (2011).

3

Mental Health Problems Kids Have

Are students mentally ill if they've been identified for special education? The short answer to that question is: not necessarily; sometimes, perhaps often, but not always. The truth is more complicated than a simple yes or no.

Mental illness and need for special education aren't exactly the same, but there's a lot of overlap. So, we can't conclude that a child qualifies for special education just because he or she is mentally ill. And we can't conclude that all of the children who receive special education—even special education for children in the federal category of "emotionally disturbed" (ED)—are mentally ill in the judgment of a psychologist or psychiatrist. They do have mental health problems in a general sense, but they may or may not meet the criteria for a diagnosis of mental illness.

> Mental illness and need for special education aren't exactly the same, but there's a lot of overlap.

Disability, Mental Illness, and Special Education

First, consider disability, which includes many difficulties that don't involve mental illness. Our colleagues and we have tried to explain the relationship of disability to special education.[1] It's not a simple relationship. Not every child with a disability needs special education. Only if a child's disability interferes with his or her *education* does he or she qualify for special education. That is, regardless of how they function outside of school, children aren't considered to have a disability *for educational purposes* unless they have problems in school *because* of their disability. The fact is that most children with a disability *do* need special education because their disability *does* interfere in some fairly obvious way with their education. But just having a disability isn't enough for the federal special education law to kick in. The federal law, regardless of its title, has had the same fundamental requirements since it was enacted in 1975. The Individuals with Disabilities Education Act, often referred to by its acronym as IDEA, was given the title Individuals with Disabilities Education *Improvement* Act (IDEIA) in 2004. When it was first enacted in 1975, it was known as the Education of All Handicapped Children Act.[2] But the law has had the same fundamental requirements since 1975, even though its title has changed over the years. Here, we refer to IDEIA as well as its predecessors as IDEA.

Children can have disabilities and mental health problems of amazing variety, and many of these problems make their education extraordinarily difficult. Consider the fact that children can have difficulty seeing, hearing, moving, thinking, behaving, talking, or any combination of these. They might have some form of autism, traumatic brain injury, or health problems. Any of these disabilities can occur not only in any combination but with different degrees of severity. So, for example, it's possible for a child to have a learning disability *and* a mental health problem, autism *along with* language and emotional or behavioral disorders, cerebral palsy *and* mental health issues—any combination of disabilities of varying nature and severity. *In fact, a child's having only a single difficulty or disability is relatively rare.*

Yes, mental health problems *can* be accompanied by *any* disability. But mental health problems themselves can also occur in a wide variety of combinations. For example, an individual might be both hyper-aggressive *and* depressed, have schizophrenia *and* an anxiety disorder, be troubled by an eating disorder *and* a substance abuse problem, and so on. In fact, it's unusual to find someone with only one mental health problem or only one manifestation of mental illness. Just consider the following cases and the multiplicity of problems a teacher or parent must deal with:

Patty

Patty's weight "yo-yos" from 105 lbs. to 180 lbs. She has had various diagnoses, including ADHD (attention deficit hyperactivity disorder), anxiety disorder, intellectual disorder (mental retardation), and schizophrenia. She appears to have a combination of many problems or disorders of a psychiatric nature. She also has vision problems and problems of physical coordination.

Jeremy

Jeremy is failing in school. He threatens other students and has been known to "punch them out." He has some relatively mild problems of physical coordination that carry the diagnosis of brain injury. Whether the brain injury was present at birth or is a result of physical abuse isn't known. He also has language problems, especially difficulty putting coherent sentences together. Many times, he seems sad or depressed, expressing a very pessimistic, almost hopeless view of his future.

It's important to keep in mind that in designing a plan of education or treatment the *individual* must be considered. Something that is appropriate in one case may be totally inappropriate in another.[3] For this reason, IDEA requires an individualized education plan for each child identified as having a disability. IDEA doesn't allow a single way of providing special education for all individuals with disabilities in the same category, much less all individuals with disabilities. So, if a school system says that *all students with X category* of disability receive a particular program or type of placement, then it isn't meeting the law's requirement of individualization. Mental health services outside special education aren't governed by special education laws, but the same general principle applies—mental health service providers must not assume that because a child has a particular type of mental health problem, a "standard" treatment is called for.

Not all disabilities affect a child's education the same way. Suppose, for example, a child has epilepsy—surely a physical disability—but his or her seizures are so well controlled by medication that the child can go to school and learn like typical children. Then, clearly, special education isn't called for at all. Or, suppose a child has schizophrenia—surely

a disabling mental illness—but the problematic delusions and halluci-
nations are so well controlled by medication that the child can go to
regular classes and learn as expected for most children of his or her
age. Then, certainly, special education isn't required. Or, suppose a
child must use a wheelchair but is otherwise unimpaired. Then nothing beyond making building(s) and classrooms physically accessible
to this child is appropriate when it comes to education. True, federal
special education law demands accessibility, but beyond that, no special program of instruction is required for a child whose only disability
is inability to walk. Keep in mind, too, that a child's disability might
get better or worse over time, so special education might be needed or
not needed at a given time, depending on the child's condition. This is
true for mental health needs as well. The need for services may not be
constant over a long period of time.

But, suppose that because of a disability a child is not able to
learn academic skills or social behavior as expected of most children.
Then special education might be required. And the details of special
education, including the *when* and *where* and *by whom* of teaching,
will depend on the details of the child's disability. Federal law—the
IDEA—requires individualized planning and selection of appropriate
educational procedures and environments to fit the child's needs. A
standard or uniform way of dealing with all disabilities, even all disabilities in a certain category (e.g., blindness, deafness, emotional disturbance, intellectual disability) is prohibited by the law. So, if a person
says something like, "Well, we offer (or should offer) only inclusion for
children with learning disabilities" or "Sorry, but we offer (or should
offer) only special classes for students with emotional disturbance,"
then they're violating or advocating violation of the federal law.

The larger question here is whether children with special mental
health needs are mentally ill. And, as we suggested earlier, we think the
best answer is that they often are, perhaps even usually are, but aren't
necessarily mentally ill. The relationship between mental illness and
special education is complex: definitely overlapping, but not always the
same. In the language of mathematics, we might say that mental illness
and special education are not an "identity" but certainly are "intersect-
ing" sets. One question we might ask is, "What percentage of children
found to have a mental illness have significant academic or behavioral
difficulties in school and are identified as having mental health problems requiring special education?" Another we might ask is, "What percentage of children identified by schools as needing special education

because of their mental health needs are found by mental health professionals to have a mental illness?" As far as we know, little or no research has been done that would answer either of these two important questions.

Even in the absence of research answering questions of overlap between the popula-

Even in the absence of research answering questions of overlap between the populations of children with mental illness and children with special education needs because of their mental health problems, we know that most of the children with these problems are neglected.

tions of children with mental illness and children with special education needs because of their mental health problems, we know that most of the children with these problems are neglected. That is, suppose that the two groups (or sets) are not overlapping at all, that they are totally different populations. Then, the evidence involving both mental health and special education is that most of the children are not served. Suppose that the two groups are the same. Then, the data lead to the same conclusion. Suppose that the groups share some overlap, that there is an intersection of the sets. The conclusion remains the same. Whether we consider the children who are diagnosed with a mental illness or those who need special education because of mental health issues, we arrive at the same hard reality: scandalous neglect.

Educational Progress and Ability to Function

School is pretty much the occupation of children, as others have pointed out. In fact, it is often their preoccupation.[4] It's really hard for a child to be judged "successful" in school when he or she is making no progress. But progress in school includes both academic and social dimensions. It's possible for one to be seen as more important than the other. For example, it's possible for a student to be doing fine academically but not socially or vice versa. This is why some definitions specify that both are important.[5]

It's really hard for a child to be judged "successful" in school when he or she is making no progress. But progress in school includes both academic and social dimensions.

Long ago, Eli Bower, an early researcher in the field of emotional problems of children in school, noted that one of the first indications of emotional problems in school is academic failure.[6] And the inability to meet the demands of school has consistently been seen as a part of most emotional and behavioral problems. For a child of school age, the ability to function satisfactorily in life includes the ability to achieve academically and behave socially as expected of most children. This does not mean that the child who functions satisfactorily will have no problems at all, simply that his or her academic or social problems are not highly unusual.

When mental health specialists refer to serious impairment of ability to function, the impairment includes functioning in school for children. Failure to make progress in school—to deal successfully with increasingly complex academic and social tasks—is often a sign of mental health difficulties and also a sign that special education is needed. Especially when the problems are severe, it's important to get special services for the child, and this might include community mental health services or special education or both.

Special Education as a Mental Health Service

Special education, properly practiced, is a rehabilitative service, not simply a way of removing students from general education.[7] Special education for youngsters who have been identified because of their emotional or behavioral problems is intended as a mental health service. Sometimes, it's the only mental health service these children get, but ideally it is in *addition* to mental health services offered by mental health providers outside of school. If mental health services are to be school-based, as some suggest, then certainly special education is part of that mental health service. Special education for aggressive behavior in elementary school may be a protective factor against later drug abuse, criminal behavior, and suicidal behavior. Nevertheless, politicians seem to feel free to "hack away" at special education programs.[8]

> Special education, properly practiced, is a rehabilitative service, not simply a way of removing students from general education.

So, what can special education provide that could be thought of as a "mental health" service? At least three things come immediately to mind: (1) help in learning the academic skills that are necessary for functioning well in the everyday context of school, (2) help in learning the social-interpersonal behavioral skills that are necessary for functioning well in the everyday contexts of school and community, and (3) help in learning the regulation of emotions and behavior that's required for personal satisfaction, social acceptance, and successful employment. That is, students' ability to function—surely one of the important goals of any mental health service—is improved when special education is appropriate because it addresses academic, behavioral, and emotional concerns.

Academic success in school is as important to children and adolescents as employment success is to adults. School is the "job" or "work" of children, and failure in school is as much a threat to children's mental health as is job failure or unemployment to the mental health of adults. Appropriate special education for children with mental health problems includes specialized instruction designed to help them acquire the academic skills they did not learn in general education—if, in fact, they have not already learned them. Contrary to popular opinion, many if not most students with mental health problems have academic deficits, and their mental health is not likely to improve unless they learn all the academic skills they can, so that they approximate the academic progress of their age peers.[9]

True, youngsters with mental health problems are more likely than the general population to have intelligence that is somewhat below average, but most of them do not have intellectual disabilities.[10] For most of these students—but not all of them—achievement within the normal range or higher is a reasonable expectation. For those who do not have academic deficits to begin with, special education is a mental health service in that it helps them keep up with their studies and achieve at a level commensurate with their abilities.

One of the hallmarks of children's mental health problems is difficulty getting along with others—not functioning well socially in school and the community. Improving the social functioning of these students is one of the major aims of special education, surely an important contribution to their mental health. Social skills that students are lacking may be taught directly. The structure and predictability of special education may be necessary to help students learn appropriate behavior. Encouragement and meaningful reward by the teacher for desirable behavior, consistent and reasonable nonviolent punishment for inappropriate behavior, and attention to the good behavior of peer models may also be part of the way in which better social conduct is encouraged in special education.[11]

Learning to deal with frustration without flying off the handle and learning to control one's emotional responses to life's typical vagaries seem easy for lots of kids, but they're often very difficult for those with mental health problems. Special education is a safe environment for students who are learning these skills at a level far below that of most youngsters their age. In general education, children are expected to have learned reasonably age-appropriate skills in expressing their anger, disappointment, frustration, satisfaction, and so on.

Special education is just that, an education that is—or should be—special.[12] It can't provide psychotherapy, and teachers can't prescribe medication. But it can, nevertheless, be an important part of the mental health services that children with mental health problems should have. If they can function adequately in general education with other mental health services, such as psychotherapy or medication or counseling, then they don't need special education. Part of the scandalous neglect of these young people is that most get neither special education nor other mental health services to help them function as well as they might.

Why Children May Not Get the Services They Need

One of the reasons many of the children with mental health needs don't get services is that there's considerable stigma attached to having mental health problems and to getting help for them. There's so much denigration of people with mental health problems that it spills over to getting help. This is most unfortunate, because it makes people not want to get services. As long as a person or family can avoid getting mental health services, the people who suggest that there is a mental health problem can be told it doesn't exist; but once a person is getting mental health services, no one can deny it. Then the people who want to demean the person who is getting the services have a basis for their denigration. They feel justified or vindicated in their judgment.

> One of the reasons many of the children with mental health needs don't get services is that there's considerable stigma attached to having mental health problems and to getting help for them.

The stigma feeds on itself. The longer one delays getting mental health services, the worse the problem becomes. The more people argue that mental health services carry stigma, the more they do. Were the reverse true—problems got prompt treatment and people considered mental health treatment desirable—people would be likely to see the advantages of early intervention, and treatment would carry less stigma. But, the way things stand now, early preventive intervention usually doesn't happen. It doesn't happen with children of any age, including those who are very young.[13]

Another reason a lot of children don't get services is that the services themselves are thought to be worthless or harmful. So, counseling, psychotherapy, or medication might be said not to "work." Of course, special education, too, is often said not to "work" as a mental health service. People find it more stigmatizing than helpful. For example, they may argue that minority children disproportionately receive special education, and thus are short-changed. But one can make the case that disproportionality has some macabre meaning only by assuming that special education is worthless or harmful or that children are mistakenly identified as needing it. The assumption with which one approaches disproportionality, if one sees it as inappropriate, must also be that emotional and behavioral problems of a given severity are randomly distributed across all ethnic groups, and that if risk factors for these disabilities do exist, they are found equally in all ethnic groups.

> Another reason a lot of children don't get services is that the services themselves are thought to be worthless or harmful.

In other areas of health—physical health problems as opposed to mental health problems—one might argue that minority children too often go untreated. To most of us, this is unacceptable. Our assumptions are that a child's health needs, physical or mental, should not be ignored because he or she is in a particular group; we treat individuals, not groups. Furthermore, we assume that: (1) children's individual needs are not often mistakenly identified; (2) risk factors affect some groups more than others; and (3) the treatment of health needs is typically effective, doing more good than harm. But when it comes to mental health services, especially special education, the arguments seem to be quite the opposite, especially that (1) minority children are often mistakenly identified for special education or other mental health services on the basis of their group identity; (2) risk factors are unrelated to identification; and (3) special education and other mental health services are not appropriate and effective in helping these children.[14] Research does not support the assumption that minority children are often misidentified for special education—unless disproportionality *per se* is taken as research evidence of misidentification—nor does research show that special education typically does more harm than good for the children who need it.[15] Moreover, recent, careful research has indicated that minority children are under-identified, not over-identified for special education, just as they tend to be in all manner of health services.[16]

Types of Disorders

There is no perfect way of classifying problems so that all ambiguity is removed and no leftover or catch-all category exists. This is likely true of almost any scientific system of classification of any type—any taxonomy. But although perfection isn't in the cards for classifying EBD, some classification systems are better or easier to understand or more helpful for some purposes than others. For example, it's entirely possible for psychiatric categories to be better than alternatives for psychiatrists, but for some alternatives to psychiatric categories to be more helpful to teachers. It's important to realize that categories or labels can't be avoided in talking about problems and that the best labels or categories are those that help people communicate most clearly.[17] We can't really talk about something without using a word for it—a label. We may be able to avoid old or familiar labels and come up with new ones, but we have to have one (a label) for something we if want to talk about it.

Psychiatric Categories

The diagnostic "Bible" for the psychiatric profession is the *Diagnostic and Statistical Manual* of the American Psychiatric Association, usually referred to as the DSM. You may want to find information about it by searching the Internet for DSM.[18]

Psychiatric categories or diagnoses are highly controversial, and although much time and effort go into the preparation of each edition of the DSM, the final draft inevitably comes in for serious, even furious criticism. The American Psychiatric Association (APA) has long recognized that some psychiatric disorders usually begin before adulthood, so there is a big or general category called something like this: "Disorders Usually First Diagnosed in Infancy, Childhood, or Adolescence" (things like learning disabilities and autism). Then, under that general category, there might be more specific diagnostic categories such as "Attention-Deficit and Disruptive Disorders" (things like ADHD and conduct disorders), "Communication Disorders" (speech and language disorders), "Elimination Disorders" (for example, enuresis), "Learning Disorders" (often called LD or learning disabilities), "Pervasive Developmental Disorders" (things like autism spectrum disorders, or ASD), and so on—and including a category called "Other Disorders of Infancy, Childhood, or Adolescence," which is a sort of residual or catch-all. Under each of these more specific categories, there will be even more specific diagnoses, each with a number (such as 307.23) and diagnostic criteria. And, depending on the category, there might be a subcategory labeled NOS (for *not otherwise specified*). In any classification scheme, there's a leftover or unspecified category, so the fact that there's a NOS category doesn't necessarily mean the classification scheme is a bad one. Remember, too, that only people with training in psychiatric diagnosis can legitimately apply DSM labels.

Then, too, there are disorders that are occasionally found in children or adolescents, such as schizophrenia and other psychotic disorders, although they're usually adult-onset disorders. In short, just because a disorder *usually* starts in adulthood doesn't mean it's *never* found in children—except, of course, dementias that come with aging or disorders *specific* to adulthood or old age. And, of course, most of the disorders *usually* first diagnosed in infancy, childhood, or adolescence *can* be first diagnosed in adulthood.

As we mentioned before, only individuals trained in psychiatric diagnosis can legitimately use the DSM to come up with a label or diagnostic category for an individual. The DSM is basically a medical guide used mostly by psychiatrists. The diagnostic category may well have legitimacy for psychiatrists in a given case but be of relatively little help to teachers or parents in deciding what they should do. The diagnosis may be helpful, particularly to psychiatrists or to those doing psychotherapy, but as guidance for those who are trying to live with the youngster or teach the child in school the DSM categories might be of comparatively little help. Parents and teachers—especially teachers—may need to find an alternative to psychiatric classification, something that they see as more descriptive of the behavior they're concerned about and more likely to help them decide what to do or how to try to help the child or youth.

Nevertheless, we also see the need for more collaborative work and better understanding of the work of the other on the part of both special education teachers and child psychiatrists. Educators need better understanding of the DSM and what the various categories mean. Child psychiatrists need better understanding of the way teachers can contribute to children's mental health and the language and classification systems that teachers might use.[19]

> We also see the need for more collaborative work and better understanding of the work of the other on the part of both special education teachers and child psychiatrists.

Alternative Classifications: Externalizing and Internalizing

One alternative to the typical psychiatric classifications is a categorical system derived from statistical (factor analytic) studies of the kind of behavior youngsters exhibit. These studies typically find that behavior can be described as falling into one of two general categories: "externalizing" or "internalizing." Another way of thinking of these two general categories is acting out or acting in.[20] These are often referred to as "dimensions" of behavior because they are derived from statistical or mathematical analyses that describe a "space" or "continuum" along which certain kinds or clusters of behavior fall.

Acting out or externalizing problems include antisocial behavior or conduct disorders—things like arguing, fighting, disrupting, and bullying. So, yes, there are more specific categories under the umbrella term "externalizing." Externalizing behaviors are hard to miss because they are, for the most part, obvious, in-your-face acts. They make other people want to get away, to avoid, not to tangle with the miscreant. It's only the unobservant teacher or parent who fails to see the typical externalizing type of behavior. True, sometimes antisocial behavior is furtive or covert, so that the youngster engaging in it is trying to "get over" or evade detection or fool people. Things like this include theft, fire-setting, vandalism, and other covert antisocial acts that harm others or destroy property. But acting out or externalizing behavior is ultimately antisocial—intended to make someone else suffer, do extra work, or escape. So, if we were to list the types of behavior that are considered externalizing, the list would include things like this:

- ◆ Aggression and related antisocial behavior (e.g., tantrums inappropriate for age, arguing, starting fights)
- ◆ Noncompliance with instructions or defiance of adults
- ◆ Breaking rules at home and school
- ◆ Hyperactivity and extreme distractibility
- ◆ Stealing
- ◆ Vandalism or fire-setting

Acting in or internalizing problems are the opposite, and there are more specific categories under the broad dimension of "internalizing." They're things like depression, social withdrawal, immaturity, and self-injury. They're the kinds of behavior that are designed to avoid interaction with others or harm oneself, not to make others want to avoid you. They may, in fact, make others want to avoid you, but that's not their *primary* intention. Depressed people may not be nice to be around, but people don't get depressed just to make others avoid them. If we were to list the kinds of behavior that are considered internalizing, the list would include things like the following:

- ◆ Excessive shyness and social withdrawal
- ◆ Avoidance of things out of extreme, unreasonable fearfulness
- ◆ Unresponsiveness to social initiations, including not interacting with peers
- ◆ Extreme unhappiness or depression, even self-injury such as cutting or suicide
- ◆ Inability to make and keep friends or build and maintain relationships
- ◆ Physical illness, pain, or complaints in response to demands or expectations

Externalizing and internalizing behavioral dimensions and the subcategories that go with them are sometimes more understandable than psychiatric diagnoses to parents and teachers. They may be more helpful in letting people who read or hear a label know what kind of behavior to expect. But they're rather general as labels, and they're most helpful only when they're accompanied by descriptions of just what a child or youth does and doesn't do that's a problem.

Multiple Problems

Regardless of the classification scheme used, it's important to understand that people of any age can have multiple problems. For example, if DSM diagnoses are considered, it's important to understand that a given individual can have more than one diagnosis, like schizophrenia *and* intellectual disability (mental retardation) or obsessive-compulsive disorder, schizophrenia, *and* a communication disorder. Or, for example, a given individual may exhibit both externalizing *and* internalizing problems, perhaps swinging quickly from one type to the other.

Multiple problems—often called comorbid problems—are common. Multiple problems are so common, in fact, that finding someone with a single problem is unusual. True, one diagnosis or category of difficulty may be dominant and the primary concern of those who provide mental health services. The focus on a particular diagnosis or category of difficulty may be understandable and helpful, but the more one knows about an individual needing mental health services, the more likely one is to find that the individual needs treatment or assistance with multiple problems.

> Multiple problems—often called comorbid problems—are common. Multiple problems are so common, in fact, that finding someone with a single problem is unusual.

Severe and Mild Problems

It's important, too, to recognize that problems in any category or of any type can range from mild to severe. In fact, everyone—or nearly everyone—has some minor problems similar to those of individuals who need mental health services. At just what point a characteristic or behavior becomes a problem is very difficult to say, and this bedevils the identification and classification of people of all ages as having emotional or behavioral disorders.

Someone's judgment is always involved, and identification and classification can't be made completely cut-and-dried. This realization allows people to argue that many of those identified have been falsely identified, that they aren't actually "over the line" and should not have been identified as having EBD. The argument is that someone made a false or bad judgment, seeing a problem that didn't actually exist or seeing a problem with an individual when the problem was (or is) actually with someone else.

One thing we need to keep in mind is that in concluding that 5 percent of the child population has a seriously debilitating emotional or behavioral problem, we're talking about children who are clearly, unambiguously over the line. They are not the kids about which reasonable people might argue (which does not mean, of course, that no one will ever argue that they're okay; some people make unreasonable arguments).

> One thing we need to keep in mind is that in concluding that 5 percent of the child population has a seriously debilitating emotional or behavioral problem, we're talking about children who are clearly, unambiguously over the line.

Cultural Differences and Emotional or Behavioral Disorders

One common argument is that a child's behavior isn't really a problem or disorder, just a difference that is okay because it is part of the child's culture, a way of behaving that is culturally normative or an insignificant departure from the expectations of the culture in which the child lives. This line of argument usually goes on to suggest that teachers or mental health service providers are not sufficiently sensitive to the child's culture and therefore mistake innocuous behavior for a disorder. Often, however, the behavior in question, even if it can be justified in some cultural settings, is not something that's okay in our society.

We might consider some possible examples, and we might remember that some of the following are or have been acceptable in various cultural groups:

◆ A boy who insists that girls can't be team captains, except for girls' teams

- ◆ A girl who makes fun of a boy's interest in dolls in kindergarten
- ◆ A student who brings a gun to school because there are guns at home
- ◆ Students who talk boisterously and laugh during a concert where they're expected to be quiet like the other concertgoers
- ◆ Students who see sexual harassment as acceptable
- ◆ Students who bully and denigrate others

Although we know that teachers sometimes mistake a cultural difference for mental health problems and one can certainly find examples of children of any cultural group who have been mistakenly identified as having such problems, there are no studies showing that such cases are typical or widespread. There is no research showing that any given percentage, even a small percentage, of minority students identified as having mental health problems and receiving special education should *not* have been identified or do *not* need the services they are receiving. Misidentification is serious, not something to be taken lightly; but we must confront two realities: (1) misidentification involves both those mistakenly identified as *having* a disorder and those mistakenly identified as *not* having a disorder, so we must consider both false positive and false negative identification and (2) careful, reliable research is needed to help us understand which problem of misidentification (false positive or false negative) is the bigger problem, why misidentification occurs when it does, and what we should do to solve the problem.

Certainly, it's possible for teachers to be culturally insensitive, and it's possible to find cases in which students have been misidentified as having mental health problems when they don't. In every human service in which judgment is required, we find mistakes of two kinds: *yes* when *no* is correct; *no* when *yes* is correct. Mistakes of both kinds are regrettable and costly to the mental health of the individuals involved and their loved ones.[21] Consider how this works for mental health problems. Mistakes of the first kind (*yes* when *no* is correct; the child is identified as having mental health problems when he or she does not) is known as a false positive. Mistakes of the second kind (*no* when *yes* is correct; the child is not identified as having mental health problems when he or she should have been) is known as a false negative. False positives have drawn the most fire from those concerned about disproportional identification of minority children, but false negatives are clearly a far more serious problem with children of *all* cultural groups, especially among at least some of the cultural groups in which disproportionate *under*-identification is the bigger problem.[22]

As we mentioned previously—and because it's extremely important, we reiterate—*all* mistakes in deciding important things about people's lives are regrettable. The objective we can reasonably have is minimizing mistakes of both kinds, realizing that fallible human beings make judgments that will sometimes be wrong. The real problem we must confront is what kind of mistake is worse, given that we're going to make one: false positive or false negative?[23] False negative mistakes lead most obviously to the scandalous neglect of the mental health needs of children with EBD. True, part of the problem of this scandalous neglect is providing no services or inadequate services for those who have been identified as having mental health needs, but an even larger problem is not identifying children who have such needs—false negative mistakes.

Notes

1. Hallahan, Kauffman, and Pullen (2018), Kauffman et al. (2018), Landrum (2017).
2. See Bateman (2017), Hallahan et al. (2018), Kauffman et al. (2018), Martin (2013), Yell, Katsiyannis, and Bradley (2017).
3. See Anastatiou and Kauffman (2011), Bateman (2017), Tucker (2010–2011).
4. See Garner, Kauffman, and Elliott (2014), Kauffman and Landrum (2018b), Walker and Gresham (2014).
5. See Forness and Knitzer (1992), Garner et al. (2014), Landrum (2017).
6. Bower (1960).
7. Anastasiou and Kauffman (2013), Evans, Weist, and Zewelanji (2007), Hallahan et al. (2018), Kauffman and Landrum (2018b), Kauffman et al. (2018), Landrum (2017).
8. See Hart, Musci, Slemrod, Flitsch, and Ialongo (2017), Levy (2017), Robinson (2004).
9. Lane and Menzies (2010).
10. Kauffman and Landrum (2018b).
11. Kauffman and Brigham (2009), Kauffman and Landrum (2018b), Kauffman et al. (2011).

12. Landrum (2017), Zigmond and Kloo (2017)
13. See Dunlap et al. (2006).
14. Harry and Klingner (2007, 2014).
15. Forness et al. (2012), Kauffman and Landrum (2018b), Kauffman et al. (2007), Kauffman, Simpson, and Mock (2009).
16. Kauffman (2010).
17. Kauffman and Anastasiou (in press); see also Gordon (2017).
18. Kauffman (2013).
19. American Psychiatric Association (2013); see also Mattison (2014).
20. See Mattison (2014). See also Kauffman and Landrum (2018b), Kerr and Nelson (2010), Landrum (2017), Walker, Ramsey, and Gresham (2004).
21. Kauffman (2007), Kauffman and Brigham (2009), Lane et al. (2012).
22. Forness et al. (2012), Kauffman et al. (2007, 2009).
23. Forness et al. (2012), Kauffman (2007).

4

Common Causes of Children's Mental Health Problems

Why do some children have mental health problems but others don't? The short answer is that we usually don't know for sure. We may suspect that certain things were causes, and some of the causes people talk about can be ruled out in some cases. But in lots of cases, if not most, we just have to admit that although we may have some idea about what the cause or causes *might* be, we just don't really know. And, unfortunately, in this context parents and kids themselves often assume that they are to blame. This makes for a lot of self-condemnation and guilt feelings that aren't appropriate, sometimes in parents, sometimes in kids, sometimes in both.

Most causes have to be thought of as possibilities or probabilities, simply because we very seldom find that a certain event or circumstance *always* causes a given problem. Some children are particularly vulnerable to some causes and seem to develop disorders under circumstances that most children seem to take in stride.

> Some children are particularly vulnerable to some causes and seem to develop disorders under circumstances that most children seem to take in stride. Others seem invulnerable to just about anything life throws at them.

Others seem invulnerable to just about anything life throws at them. And, for the most part, we really don't know *why* some youngsters succumb to potential causes and others don't. So, can we say, for example, that we know living in a dangerous neighborhood with abusive and neglectful parents is the cause of a particular child's mental health issue? No, not really. We do have very good reason to believe that such things as dangerous neighborhoods and abusive/neglectful parents are *potential* causes and that they are *risk* factors that increase the probability—the chance—that a child will have emotional or behavioral problems. We know that dangerous neighborhoods and abuse and neglect are not good things for children, that they are "risky," and we wouldn't recommend them or say we just don't care because they're just differences in kids' lives that are okay and we shouldn't be worried about them. But in the case of a particular child, we're unlikely to know for sure that the home life of the kid caused the disorder.

In most cases, we know there were probably multiple causal factors, not a single cause. It makes a lot of sense to talk about *contributing* causes—things that probably contributed to the problem, even if they aren't the only likely causes we could identify.[1]

Actual Causes and False Assumptions

The major factors that play a part in children's mental ill health are no mystery. They can be thought of as the child's (1) biological endowment, (2) family, (3) school experience, and (4) larger community or culture. All four of these major factors play an important role in shaping everyone's behavior and emotions, so it's a matter of trying to figure out what part each might play and how each of them might contribute to a child's emotional and behavioral development going wrong.

> The major factors that play a part in children's mental ill health are no mystery. They can be thought of as the child's (1) biological endowment, (2) family, (3) school experience, and (4) larger community or culture.

Before discussing each in more detail, it's important to mention some false assumptions that might mislead people into mistaken thinking about causes. The two most common false assumptions are, first, that a single cause can be found, and second, that because something is often found to accompany (go with) a disorder or happened shortly before the disorder is noticed, it's the cause.

The idea of a single cause has always fueled speculation. There is a simplicity or tidiness about the notion of a single cause that's very appealing. Mental health doesn't seem so complicated if we can point to a specific event or a single factor. If we can say something like, "Well, clearly, it's the way the parents" or "The kid obviously has the gene" or "When you have a family that models and approves of that kind of thing, then it's inevitable that you're going to get" or "It's no wonder, when you have a school like that" We like to lay the blame—all of it, or almost all of it—on a particular thing. This makes it seem that we have an explanation for the problem, and we can feel satisfied that we've figured it out. The problem is that such an "explanation" is extremely likely to be an oversimplification. But it's also extremely likely to be *partly* true and therefore difficult to dispel completely.

Almost always, if not in every case, causes work together and get very complex. This makes it extremely difficult—and probably not very helpful, at least for the particular child involved—to try to find out what started it, what was the *first* cause, the thing that kicked it off. Once the problem is launched, though, the causes are very likely multiple: one causal factor leads to others. The causes become interactive, interconnected, not easily separated. For example, academic failure and disruptive behavior in school may contribute to parental conflict and set the stage for poor parenting, which may also contribute to more school problems and community tensions, all of which may also involve elements of genetic influences and biological vulnerabilities. But biological vulnerabilities, poor parenting, and community or cultural factors may have contributed to school failure and disruptive behavior in the first place. Causes often become vicious cycles, a swirl of negative influences so inseparable that the one "culprit" can't be tagged.

There's always the temptation, too, to assume that whatever accompanies a problem must be its cause. So, if we see that poor parenting and a mental health problem co-occur—go together or are correlated— then it's tempting to assume in a given case that poor parenting *caused* the problem. It's quite true that things involving children's healthy development or developmental problems tend to go together or be correlated. For example, most of us aren't usually surprised to find that poverty, malnutrition, dangerous communities, and disabilities of various kinds are interconnected. But their correlation doesn't necessarily mean that one causes the other.

There's also the temptation to assume that something that precedes a problem is its cause. This is the old logical error known by its Latin name as *post hoc, ergo propter hoc*, or, in English, *after the fact, therefore because of it*.[2] This mistake of logic, along with the false assumption that correlation implies cause, was behind the popular 19th-century idea that masturbation caused insanity.[3] Today, we should know better than to assume that because poor parenting preceded an emotional or behavioral disorder, the cause of it was poor parenting. Unfortunately, a lot of people have bought into this kind of poor thinking. Even more unfortunately, pseudoscientists (e.g., the late Bruno Bettelheim) or persons with high public visibility have often made matters worse by greatly exaggerating the role of parents, teachers, peers, diet, vaccination, or other easily found but wrong targets of blame.

Biology

No reasonably well-informed person doubts that biological factors can and often do contribute in some way to children's mental health problems. We know that genetic factors have a lot to do with a person's physical features and physical health. We also know that virtually every aspect of cognition—including emotional and behavioral tendencies—is heritable *to some degree*. Recognizing this certainly doesn't mean that environment plays no important role in determining mental health or physical wellness. It's merely recognition of the fact that our genetic endowment is an important part of who we are physically and mentally.[4]

> No reasonably well-informed person doubts that biological factors can and often do contribute in some way to children's mental health problems.

Those who ignore biology completely live in what most scientists and lay people consider a fantasy world, what we call "la-la land" in everyday talk. It's just as remarkable for its denial of reality as the idea that biology says it all. But, what part of our physical and mental life is determined by biology and what part is determined by what we experience in our environment? We don't know exactly. Furthermore, if we're thoughtful about the answer to this question, we'll conclude that it depends on what particular feature(s) of our physical *and* mental lives. We must consider our biological *and* environmental histories. We have to consider both from the time of our conception to the present. The answer isn't easy for people who are willing to do some critical thinking about the matter.

In the early 21st century, we're not able to alter a person's genetic endowment. What you're born with is pretty much what you get in the way of genes. Of course, there are lots of treatments of biological conditions, including drugs and surgeries that might correct or ameliorate certain problems. "Gene therapy" and the alteration of genes in embryos may be on the horizon, but what relevance such developments may have for mental health is speculation at this point. Medical treatments of emotional and behavioral problems have, over the centuries, included many false starts, offered false hopes, and sometimes included pseudoscientific procedures known to have little or no benefit. Some of these pseudoscientific treatments have actually done more harm than good and delayed effective treatment.[5] However, ignoring medical contributions to the treatment of children's emotional or behavioral disorders is not wise and only deprives children and their families of help that is effective in many cases. This includes the appropriate use of medications.[6]

But, what are some of the other biological factors, besides genetics, that can come into the picture as potential causes of emotional or behavioral problems? We could think of physical illnesses and injuries; malnutrition; allergies to a variety of foods, drugs, and other substances; lead poisoning; and the mother's use and abuse of a variety of substances during pregnancy.

One biological factor we know can alter emotions, abilities, and behavior is traumatic brain injury (TBI). Although certainly not true in all cases of TBI, brain injury *can* result in mental health problems, including inappropriate emotional responses to events or situations, changes in perceptions of reality, emotional volatility, and so on. TBI is now a separate category of disability under federal special education law, but its effects obviously can include other categories of disability as well.

The fact is that the science we have to date suggests that any and all of the factors we have mentioned so far are *possible* causes of emotional or behavioral difficulties. However, in the vast majority of cases there is simply no convincing evidence that any one of them accounts for a particular child's difficulty. It's very tempting to overgeneralize and claim that one of these things (e.g., a food substance) is usually or often the trigger for difficulty, but careful analysis simply doesn't support that claim. It's also very tempting to make the logical error *post hoc, ergo propter hoc* in an individual case. That is, a great temptation in the individual case is to claim that something (for example, removal of a substance in the diet, taking a dietary supplement, taking a drug) was followed by improvement of the child's emotional or behavioral condition and, therefore, it was the cause of the improvement. The claim, "It worked for *me* (or for *him* or for *her*)" is a claim we should question. A believable claim that something "worked" has to be based on something more than the fact that improvement followed it, especially when such judgment is based on a single case—an anecdote.

Finally, we know that children are born with temperaments or typical ways of behaving and responding to various events and conditions. There are "easy" babies and there are "difficult" babies, and precisely what accounts for these differences in what appear to be biologically-based dispositions or temperaments isn't known. However, these dispositions or temperaments can set the stage for emotional or behavioral problems or make a young child relatively invulnerable to such problems. A difficult child might make it harder for parents to be warm and supportive in ways that foster healthy development. Or, parents can be so inept in dealing with a child that they turn an easy baby into a difficult child. We've known for a long time that children influence the way their parents behave toward them as certainly as parents influence their child's development.[7]

> We've known for a long time that children influence the way their parents behave toward them as certainly as parents influence their child's development.

Family

Children's families obviously affect how they feel about lots of things and how they act and react. In fact, the experience of family and the observation of family members can lead us to conclude, falsely, that the family is at the root of all emotional or behavioral disorders. Parents obviously pass their genes along to their progeny, but they also affect their children's emotions and behavior in a variety of ways—by the quality of their nurturance, their discipline, the models they provide, and so on. And to the extent that there are siblings or other relatives in the home, they also provide a social context for child rearing that undeniably affects how the child turns out.

> We must not assume that family *form* or *configuration* causes mental health problems.

We must not assume that family *form* or *configuration* causes mental health problems. For example, it's common for people to believe that anything other than two heterosexual parents, never divorced, is the only family configuration that can provide the proper nurturing and models that lead to mental health or, at least, the best one. But now we understand that single parents, divorced parents, homosexual parents, foster parents, and a variety of other family forms can provide the nurturance and models that typically lead to healthy physical and mental growth and development. That is, the *form* of the family and the personal identities of its members do not predictably lead to children's healthy development or to their having a mental health difficulty. Other factors—in fact, other *family* factors—are far more important.

Really important is the *interaction* of family members. That is, how do they treat each other? What kind of structure and discipline do the parents provide? What kind of punishment is meted out? How much supervision is provided (ranging from "helicopter" parents to those who are neglectful)? What's the attitude toward school and personal accomplishment? To what extent, and how, are children encouraged to explore and try new things? How are family members supported and encouraged? How do children respond to their parents and siblings or other family members? There are lots of other questions to ask, but these are a beginning for considering just what goes on in a family and how the interactions or social transactions between or among family members might influence emotional and behavioral development. Furthermore, any of the family structures or configurations we have mentioned can provide a good, nurturing home environment.

There's no doubt that different individuals in a given family may experience the family quite differently and that sometimes one child is treated differently from the other(s). It's quite possible for one child to be singled out for abuse or neglect or for favoritism. So, we must pay careful attention to what happens to the individual.

But it's also possible for parents to be very skilled in child rearing, unfailingly fair in the treatment of their children, and lovingly attentive to an individual child who nevertheless has mental health problems for reasons unknown. This is why it is so unfair to parents to blame them when a child has a mental health difficulty. Parents, like their children, are human beings who make mistakes. So, it's unreasonable to expect them to be perfect. And it's understandable if parents react negatively when their child behaves wretchedly or disappointingly, as all children do sometimes—but those with mental health problems more often do.

Still, we do know that some kinds of parenting are better than others and that poor parenting can increase the chances that the child will have problems. We know that parental neglect and abuse are risk factors. We know that inconsistency, in which the child doesn't know whether to expect punishment for a particular behavior, is a risk factor. Even harsh punishment that's predictable is better than not knowing whether punishment will be forthcoming, but harsh punishment (especially corporal punishment) is a parenting mistake that increases risk of mental ill health. *Authoritarian* parental discipline—in which the parents make all the rules without involving children and "lay down the law" and essentially rule the household as despots—isn't generally as good as *authoritative* discipline, in which the parent is the clear authority but is approachable.

It's virtually impossible for parents not to cause their children any trauma whatsoever at some point in child rearing, and virtually impossible for children never to frustrate if not traumatize their parents. However, some parents are extremely abusive, as depicted by Maude Julien in her memoir and Gabriel Tallent in his novel, and some parents suffer greatly because of certain actions of their children.[8] Parents may agonize over their children's mental illness, substance abuse, illegal behavior, or other social deviance. Parents and children alike can survive horrendous conditions but sustain little permanent damage and can, also, overreact to slight mistreatment or disappointment. Both adults and children vary enormously in their vulnerability and resilience. Fortunately, most families are not characterized by extremes of cruelty and trauma, but families can go awry in less extreme ways, and parental discipline can play an important role in creating problems rather than solving them.

Studies of families of aggressive children generally indicate that parents don't know how to punish their children effectively. Either they are totally lacking in rules and expectations and abandon their role as authority figures or they punish their children capriciously or viciously, acting more like despotic rulers of nations than like rational judges in a free society.[9] Reasonable reward and approval for desirable behavior and consistent *nonviolent, noncorporal* punishment for undesirable behavior are both much more effective in correcting children's behavior and much more likely to avoid contributing to a mental health problem. This means that parents should indeed be concerned about controlling their children, but they should be so without spanking, hitting, or using other physical punishment or threat of it and without lecturing or shaming.[10]

Nevertheless, parents who love their children and try their best to do what's most effective—even those who are very skilled in using punishment and rewards—are sometimes unsuccessful and find that medication may also be necessary. These parents should not be blamed or assumed to be at fault if the child continues to have problems.

Here's something to remember: The causes of mental health problems are often very complex. If the solution were simply that parents should love their children and be good parents, then few such disorders would exist.

> Here's something to remember: The causes of mental health problems are often very complex.

School

True, some children have emotional or behavioral disorders before they enter school, but it is also true that many develop such disorders after starting school. The young children with the most serious problems can be identified at an early age, and it is possible for the school to play an important role in preventing problems from becoming worse.[11]

We need to consider how schools can set the stage for problems or make problems worse. The ways a school can do this is no mystery to many people who have studied what happens to many children during their schooling, whether public or private.[12]

Schools can demand a mindless uniformity, an unnecessary and stifling conformity that serves no one well. Yes, reasonable rules and expectations are necessary, but the people who run a school can become obsessed with preservation of order and become unaware of the destructiveness of their rigidity. It isn't always easy to judge what's necessary order and universal expectation and what's not, but school personnel can squelch creativity, individuality, and harmless or healthy self-expression. Surely, this kind of over-regulation can become a reason for or exacerbate some children's emotional or behavioral difficulties.

We are not referring here to school-wide disciplinary procedures in which all the school staff agree on how to manage behavior. In fact, a good school-wide plan of discipline is really important so that teachers and students know what's expected—what's okay and what's not. All conformity is not mindless, but mindless conformity—unthinking, unreasonable, conformity that can't be explained rationally—is truly stultifying.

Sometimes too little is expected of students in school, and a laissez-faire attitude allows many children to squander their talents or never try them out. That's bad too, but the opposite can also happen. Sometimes too much is expected, setting up students for failure and making them want to avoid school. Being expected to do what you can't, whether you're a child or an adult, sets the stage for emotional and behavioral problems. None of us likes being confronted with an insurmountable challenge. In fact, it's the *just manageable* difficulty that helps us feel competent and fosters mental health.[13] In the worst of all possible school scenarios, students are allowed to squander their talents because there are low expectations for what they can do in particular areas of the curriculum, and yet there are unreasonably high expectations for them to do things they can't in other curriculum areas.

> People like to talk about having "high expectations for all students," which sounds good and noble. But having high expectations for all is not the same as having the same expectations for all.

People like to talk about having "high expectations for all students," which sounds good and noble. But having *high* expectations for all is not the same as having *the same* expectations for all. Recall our discussion of the mathematical reality of the statistical distribution that is the inevitable result of measurement. Schools will always face a range of abilities in every area of the curriculum. If students are to feel competent and stay motivated, then what's required is more than expectations. Teachers must find things students *can do now* and help them learn all they can. This requires assessing students' current skill levels and systematically increasing expectations as much as possible. In other words, children—especially those with mental health problems—need good careful, systematic instruction. Such instruction is part of creating a school environment conducive to mental health.

Schools can contribute to causing emotional or behavioral disorders by teaching students useless things or failing to teach them important things. That is, sometimes the curriculum is really not appropriate for the student being taught. By teaching things for which a student has no real or imagined use, schools can contribute to students' lack of eagerness to learn, and by failing to prepare them for life after school in ways that are important, they offer miseducation. True, what's most important to teach has always been a controversy in American public education, particularly when not all students are taught the same thing.[14] But emotional and behavioral disorders are at the very least exacerbated by a mismatch with the student's needs. For example, if a student doesn't have the needed reading skills, then trying to teach English literature to that student isn't going to be helpful and, in fact, is very likely to result in behavior incompatible with learning.

Inconsistent, capricious, or harsh discipline in schools is as likely to produce bad outcomes in school as it is in the home. The unpredictability of *some* good things may be good, but unpredictability isn't a good idea in discipline, whether at home or in school. All students, regardless of their intelligence, achievement, or demeanor, need to know what to expect when it comes to their behavior and its consequences. Teachers and school administrators who are seemingly random in their responses to students' conduct are surely flirting with disaster and certain to foster emotional and behavioral problems.

Sometimes, educators don't seem to understand that they're doing just the opposite of what they think they're doing when it comes to behavior management. They give miscreants exactly what fosters their misdeeds—attention, even if it's in the form of punishment or ridicule. Meanwhile, they ignore the kind of behavior they would like to see, often under the assumption that it should be taken for granted, or that praising or otherwise showing approval or giving any overt reward is somehow counterproductive. They get things reversed, thinking that they're going to be successful by being hard-nosed or stern and not telling students what they want or revealing any pleasure in seeing desirable conduct. They thus inadvertently produce the very problems they say they want to avoid and fail to produce the very behavior they say they want. Part of the problem here may be old notions that harsh punishment or the threat of it are effective. Part of the problem may also be the old notion that good behavior is its own reward or that it's just what's to be expected. And part of the problem may be the misinformation that reward of any kind given by an adult undermines good behavior and keeps students from developing a keen moral sense.[15]

> Students may well see emotional or behavioral problems demonstrated by others and may imitate them. They are most likely to imitate others who are more powerful than they are and those they admire.

Sometimes schools seem to encourage emotional or behavioral disorders by providing really terrible models of behavior. Occasionally, these models are provided by educators, who themselves are irritable, abusive, unreliable, depressed, or in some other way are models of maladaptive behavior. More often, models of misbehavior are provided by peers. The peers may be in either general or special education, popular or unpopular, imitated by many or only a few. The point is that students may well see emotional or behavioral problems demonstrated by others and imitate them. They are most likely to imitate others who are more powerful than they are and those they admire. Just consider the following.

***

Sarah

Sarah is a tenth-grade teacher who keeps her students in line primarily through threats, intimidation, and humiliation. She uses sarcasm liberally to belittle those who give wrong answers to questions. Her classroom environment appears orderly, but it is characterized by fear and anxiety. Somehow, she is able to explain away her bullying, repressive tactics to parents and administrators, avoiding dismissal and censure. Some parents have even expressed relief that their child finally has a teacher who will be tough on students. Administrators appreciate the fact that she handles behavior problems herself rather than sending kids to the office.

Arnie

In his fifth-grade classroom, Arnie seems oblivious to chaos. It's not just that his students are disorderly; the classroom is out of control. He seems bewildered, at best, that his students pay little attention to him, that they scream at each other, or that bullying is a frequent and overt part of his students' interactions. His behavior seems to encourage the most aggressive students to intimidate the others. He has virtually no authority in his classroom, and his students show him little respect. He explains away his ineptitude in behavior management by saying that students must be allowed to sort things out and need to learn to control themselves.

***

In spite of examples like these of inappropriate or poor discipline methods, it's unconscionable to blame teachers or schools automatically when a particular child is having difficulty. Sometimes, a very good, skillful teacher finds that a child is not responding well to excellent classroom management. Furthermore, therapies in addition to any intervention a teacher can offer, including medication, may fail to work as hoped.

Community

The community or culture in which a child is reared is a factor of considerable influence, especially as the child enters adolescence. What a child sees in the neighborhood, in social institutions, on TV, on personal electronic devices, and in movies no doubt affects his or her perceptions, attitudes, and behavior. The peer group becomes increasingly important as children get older. The community influences the child not just through the models of conduct it provides but through rewards and punishments for various kinds of behavior. In fact, various mass media (e.g., comic books, radio, TV, electronic games, Internet, movies), community institutions (e.g., churches, political action groups), peer groups (e.g., scouts, clubs, gangs), and other community characteristics (e.g., attitudes toward school, work, pregnancy, promiscuity, responsibility) have been blamed for contributing to children's emotional or behavioral disorders or failing to contribute to their resolution.

The community includes its schools, of course, but it's more than schools. It's neighborhoods, businesses, homes, churches, entertainment, institutions of various kinds (hospitals, jails, police, and so on) and even the political rhetoric heard most often. Various community influences may be contradictory or at odds—nurturing schools and churches but repressive policing, for example, or respectful policing in a neighborhood that includes deteriorating school buildings in which many educators are disdainful of students and their families.

To the extent that communities are dangerous, deteriorating environments in which children must fight for survival, they are likely to be negative influences on children's emotional and behavioral development and success in school. And to the extent that communities are nurturing, safe, and characterized by opportunity, they are likely to foster children's emotional and behavioral health. The idea that the hardscrabble environment is somehow good for children and produces real leaders who have been toughened by their struggles is a romantic notion (that the best will always overcome adversity). The notion that a good community will make identification and treatment of mental health problems unnecessary in all but very few cases is a romantic fantasy that the community can make up for everything else (is a magic mitigating factor). Both ideas—that a tough community is good and that a good community is sufficient—foster the mistaken assumption that treatment, whether it involves psychotherapy or medication, is not necessary or is relied upon too often.

We can point to many negative aspects of community life as potentially problem-causing. Likewise, we can specify aspects of communities that are likely to be good for children. But this has always been the case. The assumption that features of our society are the primary causes of children's emotional and behavioral difficulties and that children with mental health problems are being over-identified and over-medicated are popular myths with virtually no basis in fact.[16]

Myths about community safety and dangerousness are common and often are created deliberately by false information. For example, dangerousness may be over-emphasized or inflated in attempts to create fear, particularly of certain ethnic groups. Conversely, safety may be misattributed to factors that actually make homes and communities less safe, such as having more firearms (presumably in the hands of those who will use them to prevent crimes) or granting people the right to carry guns.[17]

The Tangled Web of Causes

As we mentioned earlier, it's tempting, perhaps even comforting to many, to become convinced that a particular causal factor is behind the majority of cases of emotional or behavioral disorders. Something parents said or did, the influence of the media or peer group, something that happened related to school, a risk taken with a recreational drug, a health (perhaps even mental health) problem that runs in the family—all are convenient, plausible causes for some cases. And, in a given case, it often seems that one factor or another is, if not the single cause, then the primary cause. But what we know about cause and effect should give us pause in drawing conclusions. The truth is almost always more complicated, the causes almost always more intertwined, than we like to think.

> It's tempting, perhaps even comforting to many, to become convinced that a particular causal factor is behind the majority of cases of emotional or behavioral disorders.

We like to think that we can point to a particular time or a specific incident after which everything started to go bad or things began to fall apart. This gives us a "peg," a supposed handle on dealing with difficult situations. It's like finding a specific carcinogen. For example, we're often tempted to say of a smoker who has lung cancer, "Well, he should have known that he'd get lung cancer if he smoked." The fact is, no one knows for sure *in an individual case* that smoking caused the lung cancer. We just know that smoking very substantially increases the risk (probability) of getting lung cancer. Some people smoke for many decades and don't get lung cancer; some people never smoke and get lung cancer. This is one of the things that allowed people to deny a smoking–lung cancer link for many years. Nevertheless, you can't be assured that you'll get lung cancer if you smoke, only that your chances of getting lung cancer will go way up.

Likewise, we know that experiencing harsh physical punishment by your parents increases your chances of having an emotional or behavioral disorder. Such punishment doesn't insure that you'll have a disorder; it only increases the risk. Furthermore, as in the case of respiratory disease, one factor seldom, if ever, works alone to cause an

Coming to terms with this web of causation is very difficult for many people, as unpleasant as running into a cobweb.

emotional or behavioral problem. Coming to terms with this web of causation is very difficult for many people, as unpleasant as running into a cobweb.

Cause and Treatment

Knowing the cause of a difficulty can sometimes be important, but sometimes the cause is mostly irrelevant to effective treatment. It's perhaps easier for us to understand this for physical injuries and illnesses than for emotional or behavioral disorders. For example, if a child has a broken arm, the most important immediate question is how to treat it, not whether the break was caused by falling out of a tree, a parent's angry blow, an automobile accident, a bike accident, or something else. Yes, finding out how the arm was broken may be important in preventing it from happening again, but knowing the cause of the break isn't going to change what a competent person does to treat the break; only the details of the break itself determine how it is treated. We would rather not have a physician who says, "I can't really treat this broken arm until I know exactly how it got broken." We would consider such a statement irrational and irresponsible.

Yes, usually a combination of treatments, none of which is a disproven treatment, works best. And, certainly, regardless of the cause of the problem, interventions work best when they involve both school and home.

Finding the cause of a problem can sometimes help us devise a better treatment, but it can sometimes be an excuse for delay and a cover for incompetence. In the case of emotional or behavioral disorders, we often don't know and can't find one thing that's the cause. Often, we can't be sure we've found even the primary, most significant or important causal factor. Usually, it's important to do what we can to address the problem effectively in the absence of knowing the cause. Surely, it's important to try to address the potential causes that we can, but aside from that we have to address the problem itself. Often, a combination of treatments—for example, perhaps a combination of psychopharmacology (drug treatment), behavioral therapy by a psychologist, and improved behavior management by parents and teachers—is going to be most helpful. It's tempting to put excessive faith in a single kind of treatment, just like it's tempting to assign excessive blame to a single causal factor. Yes, some treatments can be ruled out as mere superstitions or quackery. But, no single treatment works in every case. Yes, usually a combination of treatments, none of which is a disproven treatment, works best. And, certainly, regardless of the cause of the problem, interventions work best when they involve both school and home.[18]

Notes

1. Cook and Ruhaak (2014), Kauffman and Brigham (2009), Kauffman and Landrum (2018b).
2. Kauffman (2011).
3. See Kauffman (2008), Kauffman and Landrum (2006).
4. Grigorenko (2014), Johnson, Turkheimer, Gottesman, and Bouchard (2009)
5. Such treatments have included philosophical or speculative treatments with little or no basis in empirical evidence as well as abuses or misapplications (see Alexander & Selsnick, 1966; Kauffman, 1976; Kauffman & Landrum, 2006; Reisman, 1976).
6. See Forness and Kavale (2001), Forness, Walker, and Serna (2014), Kauffman and Landrum (2018b), Konopasek and Forness (2014), Warner (2010).
7. See Kauffman and Brigham (2009), Kauffman and Landrum (2018b).
8. For depictions of unusual abuse of children by parents, see Julien (2014), Tallent (2017); for reports of parents suffering because of their children's behavior, see Earley (2006), Powers (2017).
9. See Kazdin (2008).
10. See Kauffman and Landrum (2018b), Kazdin (2008).
11. See Conduct Problems Prevention Research Group (2011).
12. See, for example, Kauffman and Brigham (2009), Kauffman and Landrum (2018b)
13. Hobbs (1974), Kauffman and Landrum (2018b).
14. Kauffman (2010).
15. See Bayat (2011) for discussion of the controversy of using praise.

16. Forness et al. (2012), Kauffman and Landrum (2018b), Warner (2010).
17. Moyer (2017), Shermer (2017), Webster, Vernick, Crifasi, and McGinty (2017). The 2018 Valentine's Day shooting in a high school in Florida provided yet another example of what *The New Yorker* magazine called the disgraceful failure to protect our children (retrieved February 15, 2018 from https://www.newyorker.com/news/our-columnists/americas-failure-to-protect-its-children-from-school-shootings-is-a-national-disgrace-parkland-florida?). The shooting illustrated not only America's adolescent romance with guns and ludicrous lack of gun control but another disgraceful instance of adults ignoring deviant behavior and failing to take appropriate action concerning a child's mental health. Students and school personnel knew of the shooter's deviant behavior for a long while, but apparently no adult *insisted* on his treatment or restriction of his access to guns.
18. Reinke, Frey, Herman, and Thompson (2014).

5

Prevention Remains a Good Idea, But Is Seldom Practiced

Everybody, or just about everybody, will agree that primary prevention of all kinds of mental health problems is a good idea. That is, if we can keep these disorders from happening in the first place, virtually everyone will agree that we ought to do that. Prevention is a really good idea, an idea whose time has come ... an idea well-loved and well praised by just about everyone. Prevention as a mantra—prevention in the abstract—has no apparent enemies.

It's not the *idea* of prevention that's a hard sell. The hard sell is getting people to *do what's necessary* for prevention. Actually, the thing we're best at preventing is prevention itself—at least when the problem to be prevented is mental illness. In this chapter, we discuss what prevention is and isn't, how we might think about it, and why our society is so reluctant to do it when it comes to mental illness and emotional/behavioral problems.

Types of Prevention

At least three different levels or meanings of prevention can be described: *primary, secondary, and tertiary*. Here's a description of the three levels of prevention in a nutshell:

1. *Primary Prevention*: The problem never happens. No further action is required. And no one needs to be identified, labeled, or singled out, because everybody gets the same thing, which is designed to preclude the problem from occurring in the first place.

2. *Secondary Prevention*: The problem is caught early, and early intervention follows. Effective secondary prevention keeps the problem from getting worse and eliminates it, if possible. It doesn't keep the problem from happening, but it does deal with it right away.

3. *Tertiary Prevention*: The problem is dealt with after it's advanced, after it's been neglected for quite a while and it's really bad. The objective at this point is to keep it from becoming unmanageable or fatal.

Most often, when people think about prevention, they think about the *primary* level. Two common features of modern life are aimed at primary prevention. High, centered brake lights on cars are aimed at primary prevention of accidents; the *main* idea is to keep rear-end collisions from happening *at all*. The *main* idea of requiring helmets for bike riders and football players is to prevent traumatic brain injuries (TBI) from occurring *in the first place*.

Primary prevention is important, but it's not "the whole game" of prevention. We hope that as you read on you will understand how necessary secondary and tertiary prevention are, too. Secondary prevention, in particular, is where the real action is when it comes to mental health problems. The very disappointing fact is that, although people want to focus on primary prevention, it's often not even possible, simply because the problems have already been observed; no one can prevent what has already happened. The sad fact is that we're best at tertiary prevention. That's just the reverse of what we want. But this reality is important—when mental health is involved, we're lousy at primary and secondary prevention and spend lots of money and effort on tertiary prevention. We don't want to be awful at tertiary prevention, but we need to get lots better at primary and, especially, secondary prevention of mental health needs.

An example or two of each level of prevention might help. For example, we might consider how the various levels of prevention might apply to dental problems or to physical illness. After considering some examples of prevention in other areas, the idea of the different levels of prevention of mental health problems might make more sense.

An Example From Dentistry

Let's consider the problem to be tooth decay or cavities—dental caries.

Primary prevention means the problem never happens—tooth decay doesn't happen, cavities don't appear, dental caries aren't found. These things never start. The problem is completely averted. In dentistry, primary prevention is accomplished through such things as dental hygiene and other treatments of children's teeth. An advantage of primary prevention is that it's something everybody gets or does (or should get or do) without identifying a particular individual as having a problem with tooth decay or having a special risk for it.

Secondary prevention in this example might involve identifying cavities and filling them. And now we have to identify particular kids and teeth. We don't want to drill and fill randomly. Of course, the things used for primary prevention might be continued. But the fact is that the cavities have appeared, were not prevented, and must be addressed in a way that primary prevention alone can't handle now. It's too late to rely on primary prevention. Secondary prevention is important, and if effective secondary prevention isn't implemented things will get worse—the decay will continue unchecked. So, the secondary prevention that requires drilling out the decay and filling the tooth is really important.

Tertiary prevention in this example might be necessary if the cavity is not filled in a timely manner. It might require a crown or a root canal or both to keep the tooth from being lost completely or keep it from becoming infected and causing additional problems. It's too late now for secondary prevention; the choice now is radical treatment or letting things get out of control. True, primary and secondary prevention might still be wise for the sake of other teeth, but it's too late for those measures to address the issues with the tooth we're talking about.

A Problem Involving a Childhood Disease

We might choose any one of many different health problems for this example, but let's consider one that's easy and familiar—measles.

Primary prevention means the disease never occurs for the individual in question, so we might consider vaccination against measles just that—primary prevention, which means the child never gets measles. Furthermore, no child needs to be identified as having a special need, as the vaccination is given to all children (or, at least, should be). In the case of anti-vaxxers, the children who do *not* get the vaccine are singled out.

Secondary prevention in this example would mean the child gets the disease (catches the measles virus), but it's treated immediately. This might mean things like giving intravenous (IV) fluids, giving medications to lower the fever and ease the pain, prescribing antibiotics to treat secondary bacterial infections, and generally giving good nursing care. These are all procedures designed to keep the child's condition from getting worse. The idea is to prevent the need for the tertiary prevention that's required by complications. But keep this in mind, too: We wouldn't think of providing this kind of treatment for *all* children because they don't *all* have measles. So, we have to identify those who actually have measles and treat only those with the disease. We have to single them out if we want to help them.

Tertiary prevention in this example involves treating complications so that they are kept as few and mild as possible, disability is averted or minimized, and the child doesn't die. The complications can include brain damage, ear infections or hearing impairments, diarrhea, pneumonia, and so on. It's too late now for secondary prevention to address the problem adequately; now it's a matter of trying to keep the damage done by the disease to a minimum.

Mental Health Problems

The problems involving prevention of mental health problems and needs are quite different (or people see them in a different way).

Primary prevention involves minimizing the chances that a child will develop an emotional or behavioral disorder. Primary prevention would include things like effective teaching, wise child rearing, good nutrition, and timely health care. In schools, it would include not only good instruction but good behavior management, too.[1] These are things we can do to lower the chances that *any* child will have mental health problems, and we can do them for *all* children without identifying any as having special needs.

Remember that the idea in primary prevention is to prevent the problem from ever occurring at all. You might notice that primary prevention in all cases is something routinely given to *all* children.

There's no need to identify a particular child as needing something special or extra, simply because *all* children get the primary prevention (e.g., preventive dental care, measles vaccination, good child rearing or childcare, and effective teaching). We don't need to say, for example, that a particular tooth needs a filling, that the child needs a drug to reduce the fever due to measles, or that special behavior management is required. These aren't necessary, simply because the problems we're preventing haven't occurred. If a problem occurs—a cavity is found, measles is contracted, a mental health problem emerges—then primary prevention has failed, it's too late to rely solely on it (primary prevention), and it's important to begin secondary prevention as soon as possible so that the problem doesn't get worse.

Secondary prevention of emotional or behavioral problems can't happen until we notice a particular mental health issue. And although the secondary prevention could be applied to *all* children without labeling any as needing something special, that would be as silly as putting fillings in *all* teeth whether they have cavities or not or giving IV fluids to *all* children whether they have measles or not. It's not reasonable to give a treatment to *all* that's needed only by some. But this *does require identifying the individuals who have special needs*—and, when it comes to mental health problems, identifying the children who need secondary prevention. As far as we're able to figure out, identifying those who need secondary prevention can't be done without labeling children in some way—using a word or words, a term for their difficulty that sorts them or separates them from the rest in describing their need. We have to be able to say to each other something equivalent to "Yes, this one; no, not that one." Otherwise, we're dead in the water when it comes to doing something (remember, it's now too late to rely solely on something we do for everyone). But, remember this: This reality is so distasteful to many people that they hesitate to do secondary prevention, want to delay it, and thus inadvertently push many cases of mental health problems into the need for tertiary prevention.[2]

> It's not reasonable to give a treatment to all that's needed only by some. But this does require identifying the individuals who have special needs—and, when it comes to mental health problems, identifying the children who need secondary prevention.

Tertiary prevention of mental illness means dealing with advanced cases, ones that have become so severe and complicated that our only realistic hope is to keep from having a total disaster on our hands. Once a mental health problem gets to be so in-your-face, so obvious, so intolerable that almost no one can deny it, then people are often moved to step in with some sort of program designed to control the damage. This level of intervention is, indeed, important. But at this stage we can seldom do more than minimize damage and avoid the worst possible outcome: lifelong problems, unemployment, institutionalization, incarceration, family dissolution, serious injury, and so on.[3]

> Remember that the failure of primary prevention may well increase the need for secondary and tertiary prevention.

Remember that the failure of primary prevention may well increase the need for secondary and tertiary prevention. We see this illustrated by the example of measles. The failure of some families to vaccinate their children against measles may result in a child getting the disease and infecting others who have not gotten the vaccine.

But the problem involving prevention is very different in the case of emotional or behavioral disorders or mental illness. People often worry needlessly that because good parenting or good teaching has failed to produce the hoped for primary prevention for a given child, now *their* child will be "exposed" to a child with behavior problems and "catch" the problem. However, this "contagion" of misbehavior is very often misunderstood and overplayed. First of all, behavior is not contagious in the same way as a disease like measles. It isn't a viral or bacterial infection. It's much more like poor dental hygiene or tooth decay in its effects on others. Second, good teaching and parenting may help well-behaved children resist the tendency to imitate the misbehavior they see. Third, if an observing child begins to misbehave, then his or her behavior is very likely to be corrected quickly with good management. Finally, the failure of primary prevention is likely to increase the need for secondary or tertiary prevention only for the child for whom primary prevention failed.

So, yes, many of the principles of prevention are the same for all conditions. Nevertheless, not every principle of prevention applies to every example. It's important to see similarities that exist, but it's also important to see how analogies break down, how dental caries are different from measles, and how both of these are different from mental health problems.

The Appeal and Limitations of Primary Prevention

As we've suggested, virtually nobody argues against primary prevention; it's well loved by nearly all. Extremely few people, if any, will argue for letting children have unnecessary mental health problems. Of course, a substantial number of people may disagree about just what constitutes good mental health and how a special mental health need should be defined. Many will argue about what's necessary or inevitable or even what constitutes good child rearing or good teaching. People will disagree, too, about what good behavior management means—how to recognize it when you see it. So, right off the bat we will have some disagreement about just what it is we're trying to prevent and how we should try to do it.

However, putting those disagreements aside, nearly everybody will agree that primary prevention is a good idea. It has lots of intuitive appeal because most people will see that it will save money and frustration. But even assuming that we can agree on what to prevent and how to try, it seems pretty clear that the very best primary prevention we can muster isn't going to prevent *all* cases of whatever it is we believe shouldn't happen. It may well prevent a substantial percentage of cases that would otherwise occur, and so cut substantially the number of children needing something more than primary prevention. No matter how we try, though, it seems virtually certain that a significant number of children will slip through—will be found to have a mental health problem in spite of our best efforts to practice primary prevention. Primary prevention of mental health problems isn't so simple or so effective as primary prevention of measles. It's far more complicated. As we mentioned in a previous chapter, mental health issues are caused by many factors, and often we don't really know the cause.

> We can conclude this about primary prevention: It's necessary, but it's not sufficient.

So, yes, primary prevention is a good idea. Yes, we should do it. Unfortunately, no, primary prevention alone is not going to be enough. We can conclude this about primary prevention: It's necessary, but it's not sufficient. We might also note this: When people say that we should "catch them before they fail" they're almost always talking about primary prevention of academic problems, not emotional or behavioral issues. And primary prevention is something done for *all* kids or in *all* cases, without singling out those who have already _____ (e.g., failed in some way academically, exhibited unusual behavior problems). Once we see academic failure or an unusual behavior problem, it's too late to catch it before it happens—too late for primary prevention alone. This may seem logical or completely obvious to you, but it often isn't apparent when people talk or write about prevention of mental health issues or other problems leading to the need for special education or other mental health treatment.

Chances With Secondary and Tertiary Prevention

Once a mental health problem has been noticed, it's clear that primary prevention didn't work in this instance and secondary prevention is the proper focus—trying to keep the problem from getting worse, and eliminating it, if possible. The earlier the problem is noticed and addressed, the better the chances of reducing or eliminating it. The longer the problem goes untreated, the worse the chances of doing so.

> The earlier the problem is noticed and addressed, the better the chances of reducing or eliminating it. The longer the problem goes untreated, the worse the chances of doing so.

Early identification and intervention are possible, but both are problematic and relatively seldom practiced for reasons we discuss further.[4]

Unfortunately, the typical response to a mental health problem is to let it go until it gets really bad, obvious, intolerable, and difficult to treat or overcome. The delay is rationalized in various ways that we discuss further. But the point here is that disorders often get to the point that the only real hope is to keep them from overwhelming the family, school, or other agency. Often, whatever is done is done under duress, perhaps with pressure from juvenile justice, social services, or the department of mental health, often under emergency conditions. Decisions made in emergencies are often not particularly good ones, and the outcome is often little more than temporary containment of the problem.

Perhaps actions speak louder than words, to use an old cliché. What we do to make prevention a reality is very little, although we praise the idea to the sky. It's difficult, if not impossible, to admit the discrepancy between our words and our actions unless we do a very careful analysis of why people say one thing and do another. So, now we discuss some of those reasons that people are hesitant to do what actually needs to be done.

Developmental Optimism

Generally, we think of optimism as desirable and likely to help people overcome adversity. And in many situations, if not most, that's true. But, depending on just what one is optimistic about, the degree of one's optimism, or the action one takes based on an optimistic forecast, it's possible that the optimism isn't helpful and may, in fact, be quite the opposite. It's usually good to be optimistic about children's development, and many children, if not most, do have some problems, including problems in regulating their emotions and behavior. Most of them do manage to right themselves and "outgrow" their problems or get over them to become reasonably healthy adults. Nevertheless, a substantial number don't and have chronic problems.

Optimism about the emotional and behavioral development of children, especially in light of the fact that most children have some emotional and behavioral problems and get over them, often leads people to say to themselves for too long, "Yes, I know he's having some problems now, but I think they'll pass," or "Yes, I know she's going through a really rough patch right now, but I think she'll outgrow it," or "Sure, this kid looks like she (or he) has a behavioral problem now, but all kids go through this, and I think if we just don't label the kid and get all bent out of shape everything's going to be all right." This kind of developmental optimism often seems justified, and it's hard to know when a prediction that everything's going to be fine is accurate. It's very difficult to know when a prediction that things will be fine is wrong, especially in the earliest stages of what may turn out to be a chronic disorder. But, if the optimistic view is wrong, then we've missed a chance for early identification and intervention.

Denial of Disorders

Denial of whatever we'd rather not acknowledge for any reason is both easy and common. Denial of a drinking problem is what keeps alcoholics and their enablers out of treatment. Denial of eating and exercise problems is what helps both the morbidly obese and the anorexic maintain their weight problems and not change their eating and exercise habits. Denial of the link between smoking and ill health made cigarette manufacturing and sales very profitable for decades, and it still allows cigarette companies to stay in a profitable business. We could give many examples, but the point is that denial of EBD is no exception. Denial of a mental health issue is often easy until the possibility of secondary prevention has passed and tertiary prevention is the only real hope.

Denying that there is a problem does give us a "breather." And immediate relief is appealing enough to help explain why denial is a popular option. It seems to "work," at least temporarily, sometimes for a long time. It doesn't cost anything (except that the problem may be allowed to get worse and be harder to treat later—but the problem *could*, and sometimes does, resolve itself). In a sense, denial is a calculated risk, a bet that the problem will not have to be confronted. This saves the immediate expenditure of energy, the necessity of talking about (and thereby labeling) a problem. The long-term consequences may be either horrible or negligible. For certain, though, the immediate consequence of relief from having to deal with the problem is much to the liking of most people.

Sometimes people recognize a problem but choose to do nothing. This might be considered a partial denial—of the fact that *treatment* of the problem is necessary. Often, the treatment is said to be worthless or at least highly questionable. Sometimes, even the desirability of treatment is acknowledged, but there is no action, no carry-through on actually getting treatment. This is another kind of partial denial, the kind of do-nothingness that sometimes drives professional caregivers to distraction. It's the kind of denial that puzzles and frustrates many people in all of the health care professions.

Fear of Mistakes

The problem of prevention would be no real problem at all—prevention would be a real "piece of cake"—if we didn't have to worry about mistakes. What makes prevention a problem is that we often don't know for sure what's going to happen. We don't know whether the emotional or behavioral problem we see is going to get better or worse. Forecasting the weather is easier than predicting a mental health problem. But, if the weather forecast is wrong, usually it's no big deal to most people (for some, though, it's something that makes a huge difference, especially if the forecast is for severe weather). The forecast for mental ill health is a bigger deal the more certain it is that the child is headed for trouble.

Deciding whether to ignore an emotional or behavioral problem or do something about it is almost always a huge deal to the people involved. Make a mistake either way, and somebody's going to suffer. And they may suffer a great deal. So, we return to our previous discussion about what kind of mistake is worse: doing something when we shouldn't have (a false positive) or *not* doing something when we should have (a false negative). The designation *false positive* and *false negative* gets confusing, so here's something that might help. Remember, we're talking about mistakes, so it's just a matter of which one is worse; a *yes* answer to the question that should nave been answered *no*; or a *no* that should have been a *yes*). Notice that we're talking in both cases about being wrong (hence, the *false* designation); the cases in which we *don't* make mistakes are known as **true** *positives* and **true** *negatives*.

Decision: **Yes**, child has a mental health disorder; but that's
  wrong—**False Positive**
Decision: **No**, child does not have a mental health disorder, but
  that's wrong—**False Negative**

Usually, if the cost isn't considered excessive, or if the outcome of one kind of mistake is clearly worse than the other, then we hedge our bets on the side of safety. Consider some safety features of automobiles (e.g., seatbelts, air bags). We have these because the cost of a false positive is relatively small (that is, the cost of having these devices—effectively deciding that yes, we will have a wreck when we're not going to—is comparatively small), and the cost of a false negative is horrific (that is, the cost of *not* having these devices to protect us—effectively deciding that no, we're *not* going to have a wreck when we *will* have one—is very high). Or consider the cost of a false positive in the legal system—falsely convicting a person. In the legal tradition, we'd much rather a guilty person go free than falsely convict a person, so we prefer the false negative (no, not guilty, but we're wrong). In law, prefer a wrong *no* to a wrong *yes*. Or think of a physician. The worst terror for a doctor is usually a false negative (e.g., missing and not treating a disease), even though a false positive (diagnosing and treating a disease that didn't exist) is no joke and can have horrible consequences. Whether we'd rather see a false positive or a false negative decision depends a lot on what we see as the consequence of making a mistake. In medicine, for example, we surely don't want a false positive when deciding to amputate; we certainly don't want a false negative when the disease is AIDS.

So, really, when it comes right down to it, we have to decide which is the worse kind of mistake to make when we're wrong about mental health and mental illness: false positive or false negative? We'd like not to make mistakes, and any mistake will disappoint if not haunt us. But which is worse in the case of a child's emotional or behavioral difficulty: letting something go when we should have acted, or stepping in when we should have let it go? Unfortunately, we often have to guess which way to go. Our guesses may be well-informed, but sometimes they'll be wrong.

In our society, we seem clearly to prefer false negative to false positives when it comes to children's mental health problems. That is, we'd sooner say, "Naw, don't worry" and later be found wrong than say, "Gosh, we'd better get on this problem pronto" and be wrong because, actually, everything's going to be okay. When we look at the data, it seems exceedingly clear that we moan and groan about false positives when it's the false negatives that far more often come back to bite us. We're more afraid of someone considering us overzealous or calling us a "worry wart," a "nervous Nelly," or a "bleeding heart" than we are about someone saying, "I told you so!" or asking, "Why didn't you *listen* to me?" or "How'd *that* one get past you?" The false negative can be more easily explained as a matter of wanting to protect the child's or family's privacy or stop the intrusion of government into people's lives or save resources and money until the problem has gotten out of hand or is obvious to everybody.

Labels and Stigma

As we mentioned above, early intervention—secondary prevention—demands identification of the individual child, labeling, saying, "Yes, this one." There is no way around labeling—unless, of course, you're just going to keep the existence of the problem to yourself and not talk about it to anyone else (then only *you* have identified the child, and you've only done the labeling in your own mind). But as soon as you or someone else talks about the disorder, the child has a label. It really is as simple as that—communication requires a label. And, if you just keep the observation of the problem to yourself, then prevention is virtually impossible because only you will be able to do anything about it.[5]

Yet labeling is one of the greatest objections to identifying children with mental health disorders. People worry that naming the problem will make it worse. They think that as long as the problem isn't talked about or is talked about in some sort of code that softens the language describing it, things will be better. For example, they might think it's better to speak of "mental health challenge" rather than "mental health disorder." So, parents or psychologists or teachers might be horrified at the prospect of saying that a child has a *disorder*—or at least object to or be very hesitant to say it. Yes, caution is wise, but someone can be overly cautious or use caution to delay effective treatment.

Perhaps the primary reason people object to labeling is that labels related to mental health issues are thought to be extremely stigmatizing. Few people are completely unconcerned about others knowing that they have been diagnosed with a psychiatric illness or emotional/behavioral problem—or that their child has been. And most people are very reluctant to have more people than absolutely necessary know that they are, or their child is, receiving psychological or psychiatric treatment or is receiving special education. True, people are normally and rightfully concerned about their privacy and are often discreet in talking about their or their own or their child's physical health. But they are even more reluctant to talk openly about mental health problems and their treatment because such problems and the need for their treatment is thought to be shameful, to reveal a personal weakness or fault, to carry a far worse stigma than problems of physical health.

Ironically, the more people obsess about the stigma of labels, the more stigmatizing the labels become. It's often difficult to overcome stigma, but it's also rather clear that the more openly a problem or condition or choice is talked about without condemnation, the less the stigma attached to it. By being reluctant to talk about mental health and mental health problems, by repeating the conventional wisdom that such problems and disorders are shameful and it's damaging to name them, people inadvertently increase the negative attitudes that already exist.[6]

Other Consequences

Unfortunately, labeling and stigma are not the only consequences we must consider. Of course, there are the consequences of false identification, which can be unnecessary worry and lost opportunities. These are not trivial issues. However, in weighing serious negative consequences, those resulting from false negatives are a far bigger problem, not only because false negatives far outnumber false positives but also because worry, stigma, and lost opportunities are compounded. The disorders not addressed grow worse and more intransigent; the consequences of doing little or nothing grow more dire as the disorders grow worse. Chances dwindle for success in education, gainful employment, stability in human relationships, and personal satisfaction.[7]

Cost

We do not have many good cost/benefit studies of special education and other mental health services. We do have a few, and as we mention in the next chapter they suggest the cost of doing nothing is way higher than the cost of effective early intervention. It's also clear that jail costs more per individual per year than does school and that academic and social success in school are more likely to lead to a low need for social services of various kinds later in life. So, picking up problems early in school and addressing them in ways that help youngsters become more successful is a good bet as an approach to prevention. Will we successfully avert jail for every child identified and served early by special education or mental health? Of course not. But our batting average is likely to be high enough to save money for taxpayers and avoid much personal trauma (for both those identified and their families, teachers, or victims). Perhaps the old bromides apply, that "grease is cheaper than machinery" (the literal statement could be interpreted metaphorically to mean that prevention is cheaper than addressing disasters after the fact) and "an ounce of prevention is worth a pound of cure."

In an era of great concern for cost saving, we might think that prevention is a winning idea. There is one huge problem: Prevention requires spending money *now* to save money *later*. Regardless of any logical argument about long-term cost saving, the order of the day is to cut budgets and save money *now*. So, prevention typically dies with phony praise.

Notes

1. For an example of prevention practiced on a school-wide basis, see Lane, Kalberg, and Menzies (2009), Lane et al. (2012).
2. For further discussion of prevention of emotional or behavioral disorders, see Kauffman (1999, 2011, 2013, 2014), Kauffman and Landrum (2018b).
3. Walker et al. (2004)
4. See Dunlap et al. (2006), Kauffman (2013, 2014). See also Samuels (2018).
5. Kauffman (2013, 2014), Kauffman and Badar (2013).
6. See Jamison (1995), Kauffman (2011).
7. Walker et al. (2004); see also Hart et al. (2017) for evidence that early special education may be a protective factor rather than a risk factor for later problems.

6

What We Should Do

Nearly anyone who understands the scandalous neglect of children with mental health problems will ask, "Well, okay, so what do you suggest we do about it?" We suggest "biting the bullet" by advocating more effective special education and related mental health services for a far greater percentage of the child population.

We refer to biting the bullet because we, and anyone doing what we suggest, will likely encounter very strong resistance. We are likely to be called uncomplimentary names for what we recommend. Virtually all of those who object to what we say, and those who call us names, will claim, for obvious reasons, that they really want to prevent mental health problems and they want to meet the needs of those in our society who actually need help because of a mental illness.

> Highly predictable objections to identification and treatment of mental health problems will be raised, especially the following: violation of privacy, creation of stigma, ineffective treatment, and prohibitive cost.

Nevertheless, highly predictable objections to identification and treatment of mental health problems will be raised, especially the following: violation of privacy, creation of stigma, ineffective treatment, and prohibitive cost. These are not the only objections likely to be raised, but they are among the most predictable. We remind readers that problems cannot be addressed until they are identified and that these are problems of particular individuals, who must be identified. And identification starts with measurement—comparison of what we are concerned about with what we would like to see.

We summarize some of these predictable objections, the arguments against identification and intervention that are most certain to be raised. Then we make our counterarguments to those predictable objections.

Arguments Against Intervention and Counterarguments

So far, the arguments against intervention have carried the day. They have convinced most people to do very little or nothing about the problems they see. So, as a society, we delay until intervention is less effective and costs more than if we had intervened earlier. We explain the predictable arguments against earlier intervention and, immediately following each predictable argument, we launch our counterarguments.

Violation of Privacy

The Predictable Argument
Violation of privacy is one issue certain to be raised by those who see schools as institutions that should limit their interest to academic matters. This argument gains steam as hackers steal personal information stored on electronic devices. Surveys, ratings, and scales designed to identify those who need help for emotional or behavioral problems will surely be cast as intrusive and dangerous—both because they encourage introspection and judgments of others and because of the possibility of theft of personal information. Interventions will be portrayed as off-target and as government meddling in what should be a private, family concern, particularly if the school is a public institution or if the intervention is publically funded. In some cases, people will suggest that the real problem is bad parenting advice from psychologists and others and claim that the best solutions are (1) inducing

shame and guilt for misbehavior, (2) expelling those students who are chronically disruptive, (3) making school disruption a matter for the police and courts to handle, and (4) allowing market forces to work. People will make comments like, "Well, actually, what teachers do doesn't matter much because parents' choices and market forces will ultimately determine what works and what doesn't."[1] Then, according to this argument, teachers will use the instructional programs and behavior management strategies that reliable research shows actually work, or work best.

Counterarguments

The violation of privacy argument strikes at the first step in intervention: measurement of mental health. We might also note that, so far in the history of education, parents and market forces have not brought us education that's based on scientific principles and has been demonstrated by scientific studies to work.[2] Parents of children with mental health problems are, in many cases if not most, tired of privacy arguments that end up denying their children effective treatment.[3] But, of course, the parents who speak out on this issue are likely to be those who have struggled for years with their children's disorders, not those involved in *early* intervention. Much more difficult will be obtaining the support of parents of children whose difficulties are less obvious and of shorter duration. However, extending services to more children whose problems are just emerging is necessary if prevention is to become more than popular blather.

The right to privacy—including the right to reject treatment for illnesses, physical or mental—is a deeply held American tradition.[4] One consequence of this concern for privacy or individual agency is the denial of diagnoses and rejection of treatment of minors by adults. In the case of mental health problems of children, this is very often used not only to condemn screening but to reject all types of early identification and intervention. Casting the privacy concern as more important than any other does this: It effectively kills prevention.

The hacking of electronic devices to obtain personal information is a legitimate concern. However, such hacking is motivated most often by the determination of criminals to obtain financial information or data that make fraud possible in financial transactions or that can be used to blackmail someone. These motives would seldom or never encourage hacking into mental health data regarding children or adults unless mental health problems and their treatment are considered damning secrets. In future years, mental health treatment may be better accepted, becoming as easily accepted as treatment of physical health problems, and lose some of the stigma that makes people want to be secretive about it. Moreover, as cybersecurity becomes a greater issue, electronic devices and their data are likely to become increasingly secure.

The right to privacy may be invoked in self-destructive ways. When arguments of right to privacy stymie efforts to provide helpful services, then the privacy argument could be interpreted to discourage identification and treatment. In fact, the privacy argument could be interpreted to discourage or preclude intervention because identification and treatment are private matters. Some would argue that parents have rights that include their decisions not to educate their child, not to vaccinate their child against highly communicable diseases, not to allow their child to receive medical treatment, or to treat or not treat their child in other ways that some may consider abusive (this is often an issue in child discipline) or by declining interventions designed to promote health. We think these parental rights are not absolute.

When the right to effective treatment of children's mental health problems is weighed against the right to privacy, the argument for treatment should, in our opinion, carry the day. The potential benefits to the child and to the larger society can't be ignored or made secondary to other concerns. And justifiable and effective treatment can't be offered in the absence of assessment of the problem and identification of the individual. Yes, privacy is an important issue, but it is not, we feel, as important as the issue of effective treatment and the public good. Privacy is perhaps an issue specific to the problem being addressed, and prevention of children's mental health difficulties is, in our opinion, an issue in which the privacy argument should not be allowed to preclude the actions required for prevention.

Creation of Stigma

The Predictable Argument

Stigma is certain to be raised as an argument not to identify or intervene. The stigma that inevitably accompanies being identified as having a mental health problem—being labeled or having one's problem labeled—and receiving treatment (such as special education, psychotherapy, or medication) will be described as horrific and probably worse than the consequences of ignoring the problem.

As long as the problem can be denied, its stigma can be denied, too. However, the manifestation of the problem may carry its own stigma; but the argument will be that labeling the problem will make the stigma worse, and any benefit of treatment of the problem is unlikely to outweigh the disadvantage of the stigma that goes with identifying and labeling it.

Counterarguments

Certainly, stigma does accompany the treatment of problems, but we must consider whether stigma is best addressed by (1) denying or not naming problems and avoiding treatment or (2) educating the public about problems and their treatment.[5] Nevertheless, concern for the stigma that goes with being identified and talked about is sure to be raised as an objection when mental health is the issue.

But, we must consider the fact that problem behavior carries its own stigma, and we must ask whether insult is added to injury by (1) allowing problem behavior to go untreated, often resulting in inappropriate punishment or (2) increasing the level of punishment or making misbehavior a matter of police citation and court action. Stigma isn't as likely to be created, in our opinion, by attempting to find effective, nonpunitive ways of treating misbehavior.

> The idea that stigma will be avoided if we just don't label a problem (i.e., don't name it, don't talk about it, at least not using understandable language) is very persistent.

The idea that stigma will be avoided if we just don't label a problem (i.e., don't name it, don't talk about it, at least not using understandable language) is very persistent. The idea that stigma comes from the words used to describe it rather than from the perception of the phenomenon itself has a certain appeal, probably because it's partly true. People can attribute demeaning intention to almost any word, and certain words clearly convey negative meanings. But, we must recognize two realities: (1) changing a word doesn't change the phenomenon to which it refers and (2) any word or phrase we use as a substitute because we think it's less demeaning can and will be used as an epithet, a way of denigrating others. Sometimes a word may need to be avoided or changed. "Idiot" and its variants have become slang for unreasonableness, but terms related to intellectual disabilities have rightly changed. No one today would publish a book called *Idiocy and Its Treatment by the Physiological Model*, a title published by the French-born American psychiatrist, Edouard O. Seguin, in 1866. Seguin did pioneer treatment of individuals now said to have intellectual disabilities. His terminology was appropriate in his day, when the common street language was "fool." Certainly, what we might call street language needs to be avoided—calling a kid with mental health problems or abnormal behavior a "jerk," "psycho," or "wacko," for example.

Often, however, it's better to help people understand the phenomenon to which the word refers than to change the word. The creation of stigma is often a misguided argument that delays or denies helpful services.

Ineffectiveness of Treatment

The Predictable Argument

People may say that they simply don't believe in the identification and treatment of mental illness, often explaining that in their culture or in their community mental health problems are (or should be) dealt with differently (i.e., not by medication or cognitive-behavioral therapy, for example). Only the most extreme cases, they suggest, merit intervention beyond that routinely provided by the community, even if the community offers little or nothing identifiable as treatment. The routine response to mental illness in their community, they may suggest, is tolerance for difference, support from an extended family, and encouragement of normal family and community activities. These, they may argue, are traditional and sufficient.

> The seemingly innocuous, loving community care described by many advocates of non-intervention—as opposed to what are described as culturally insensitive, intrusive, or coercive treatments—too often appears to be imaginary.

Counterarguments

The seemingly innocuous, loving community care described by many advocates of nonintervention—as opposed to what are described as culturally insensitive, intrusive, or coercive treatments—too often appears to be imaginary. Homelessness, imprisonment, and even death are often the consequences of a hands-off attitude toward treatment.[6]

Streets and jails do not have to become the predominant habitats of adults with severe mental illness, which they are now. But if that is to change, then a substantial change will be required in attitudes toward the emotional and behavioral problems of youngsters, including a change in the way these problems are handled in schools.

Another factor that keeps people out of treatment is high-profile horror stories of treatment gone bad, or the outright abuse of residents in treatment facilities, or abuse at the hands of ostensible therapists.[7] Such horrors occur far more frequently than anyone but a misanthrope would like (most of us would prefer that they never, ever occur), but they are neither typical of mental health treatment nor as common as the abuse and neglect of people with emotional or behavioral problems who are *not* receiving treatment.[8] Perhaps this is much like the fear of flying created by media attention to air disasters or near disasters, although auto travel is much riskier. Perhaps it is somewhat like the fear of surgery created by reports of surgeries gone terribly wrong—horrible, indeed, but rare.

True, horrid things sometimes happen, and treatment of emotional or behavioral problems is sometimes ineffective. Anecdotes of horrors and failures stoke resistance to helpful intervention and provide fodder for arguments that treatment is futile.

The more important fact is that effective treatment for mental health problems is readily available. As we describe further, one treatment based on behavior that can be seen is called cognitive-behavioral therapy (CBT). It is aimed at both behavior and thoughts the patient has. Sometimes, pharmacological treatment and CBT have been used in combination. Both medication and CBT have been shown to have beneficial effects with many types of mental health problems.[9] Such treatments have been found successful both in homes when parents are involved and in classrooms with teachers serving as the providers of treatment.

Unjustified Cost

The Predictable Argument

Immediate cost, not long-term cost, is what motivates most lawmakers and most voters. The cost of treatment for mental health problems is often not paid by health insurance, so people seeking treatment must often pay for it out-of-pocket. However, including such treatment under insurance coverage, regardless of the insurer, drives the cost of insurance up. And treatment is anything but free of cost, so expanding the number of individuals receiving treatment obviously requires additional expenditure.

One argument of those who are primarily concerned about reducing the cost of public services is that special education and related mental health services are a waste of money because they don't work. The criteria for "work(s)" are often unclear or unrealistic. For example, a service might be said not to "work" because it fails to bring the recipient clearly or permanently into what is considered the normal range of behavior. A more realistic criterion of "works" might be that the service results in a better or higher level of functioning than the recipient would have attained with no treatment, delayed treatment, or an alternative treatment.

Counterarguments

Of course, nontreatment by mental health professionals will mean other costs. Prisons cost a lot of money. The cost of prison per person rivals or exceeds that of the cost of hospital care. And prisons have become the abode of many people with treatable mental illness.[10] Fewer people would likely be incarcerated and more people would likely be gainfully employed were mental health services, including hospitalization for those who need it, readily available. But conservative political views apparently tend to be associated with even lower rates of identification of the mental health issues of children and youth than is typical.[11] Thus, ostensible concern for lowering cost by denying services may actually have the effect of increasing the eventual cost of responding to social deviancy.

In fact, economic analyses suggest just the opposite of cutting effective services—if the concern for cost is saving money in the long term rather than spending it foolishly in the short term. Simply put, long-term follow-up programs of early intervention for young children at high risk show about a 2:1 ratio of long-term savings. That is, spending money on effective early intervention saves about $2 for each dollar spent to fund the program.[12] The savings of government expenditures include increased tax revenues from those who are employed, decreased welfare participation, reduced outlays for various types of services (e.g., special education, emergency medical care, stays in homeless shelters), and lowered criminal justice costs (e.g., for courts and imprisonment).

Purely economic costs don't take into consideration the reduction of anxiety and suffering with effective early intervention. Here's a summary statement published in 2004:

> Across the few rigorous economic evaluations done to date, the conclusion that government savings ultimately exceed costs for early intervention programs means that public investment in these programs can be justified. There are additional monetary benefits to society for early interventions, as well as intangible benefits (i.e., well-being) that improve the value of such investments.[13]

Even if people aren't persuaded by arguments that the well-being of others should sway public policy, purely economic motives should move them to support effective early intervention programs. True, the savings are long-term, not immediate. But, only those who must have immediate gratification can argue in favor of the short-term cut over the long-term saving. True, also, that the ratio of saving to expenditure may fall at some point as risk for mental health disorders decreases because we get better at primary and secondary prevention.

Two points are worth consideration here. First, even if the ratio of benefit to cost falls from 2:1 to 1.1:1.0, the expenditure is wise. Only if the cost/benefit ratio is equal to or less than 1:1 can someone possibly argue that the cost of a program is unwise on purely economic grounds. And only if the cost/benefit ratio is less than 1:1 (i.e., benefits are less than cost) *and* there are no intangible benefits can one argue against intervention on moral grounds.

Effective and Ineffective Treatments

Some treatments are more effective than others. Some are highly effective in most cases and virtually worthless in others. Some are virtually worthless or worse in nearly all cases. The best evidence of effectiveness derives from scientific tests. The least reliable evidence is testimonial—an individual's experience or personal recommendation. True, experience and recommendation may be given for effective treatments, but when such testimony is not consistent with evidence derived from scientific tests it can be highly misleading. To the best of our knowledge, treatments based primarily on unseen things are least effective.

Treatments Based on Things Unseen

Some treatments are based primarily on things that can't be seen directly: internal emotional states, unconscious motivations, thoughts, or self-talk, and so on. Traditional Freudian psychoanalysis, for example, involves a lot of interpretation of the *meaning* of behavior (not the behavior itself) and has been largely abandoned because so little evidence supports it. However, treatments such as cognitive-behavioral therapies involving what people think and feel as well as how they actually behave have a much better track record.

What people think about things and how they are feeling are surely important in helping them. This is true of youngsters as well as adults. We can't ignore this. Nevertheless, treatments based *solely or primarily* on thinking and feelings or interpretations of behavior haven't been very successful. Thoughts and feelings are extremely hard to change without paying attention to behavior, too. No wonder the most successful treatments are those that pay attention both to behavior and what's going on in a person's head, that you can't see directly.

Importance of Evidence-Based Treatments

The matter of the base of evidence underlying any treatment is important. Treatments supported by little or no evidence—by testimonials and data that most scientists would find very questionable or shaky, if not misleading—are extremely likely to result in eventual disappointment. That is, claims that they "work" are probably false. But the peddlers of treatments lacking an evidence base often claim their treatment has one. They often complain that the scientific community has conspired against them, that the evidence is being suppressed, or that science is simply incapable of testing their treatment. Sometimes they claim as "scientific" evidence something that will not pass a reasonable test of skeptics.

"Evidence-based" has become a mantra and a claim that often can't be substantiated. This is in part because of federal laws and popular demands for "evidence-based instruction." Unfortunately, claiming that something is evidence-based does not make it so. A real "breakthrough" in education and mental health treatment is extremely rare, and most claims that a revolutionary or breakthrough treatment has been found are eventually debunked. Reliable scientific evidence is typically accumulated only over a period of years and with considerable effort. And before a claim of an evidence base for any teaching, behavior management, or therapy procedure can be substantiated, it has to be tried out and the results must be replicated (i.e., duplicated) by others who did not devise it. This takes patience, money, and examination by skeptics. Yet, treatment supported by the best scientific evidence we can muster is critically important to success.[14]

> Reliable scientific evidence is typically accumulated only over a period of years and with considerable effort.

Treatments Based on Behavior and Cognition

Some treatments—often special education, sometimes medications and psychotherapies too—are behavioral. "Behavioral" means based primarily on the behavior someone can see, the way the child acts. Purely behavioral treatments are relatively unconcerned with "hidden" or unconscious motivations. They usually involve defining and counting specific problematic acts that are to be decreased and specific desirable acts that are to be increased. The basic idea is that the behavior itself (either the presence of it or the lack of it) *is* the problem, and that if the child's behavior becomes consistently appropriate, then the problem is solved. For example, the problem might be defined as hitting others, as arguing, as not completing homework, or as not obeying parents' instructions. Then, if the child stops hitting or arguing (or does so much less frequently) or does homework or obeys parental instructions (or does so much more frequently) the problem is seen as resolved.

Behavioral treatments usually involve changing what happens just before or just after the behavior that is problematic. What happens just before the behavior might be called *antecedents*; what happens just after the behavior might be called *consequences*. So, changes in behavior might be tackled by altering the antecedents of behavior—what happens *just before* or the context in which it occurs. Or the problem behavior might be changed by altering the consequences of behavior—what happens as a result of it or *right after* it. Of course, both antecedents and consequences could be changed in attempts to change the youngster's behavior. A competent behavior therapist will examine the circumstances of misconduct (the antecedents) *and* the effect that misconduct has, what it produces as a result or its consequence.[15]

For example, a child's following instructions might be improved because the parent or teacher becomes aware that an antecedent needs to be changed. Perhaps when the parent or teacher is careful to give one instruction at a time, to give it clearly as a command, and to make sure the child is paying attention before giving it, then the child typically follows instructions. Or, perhaps the consequences of failure to follow instructions need to be changed. The consequences of not following instructions might be that the child is ignored (essentially, there is no definite consequence). Alternatively, the consequence of not following an instruction could be a bonanza of attention in the form of criticism, reprimand, or arguing. The child might follow instructions far better when the teacher or parent provides praise or another form of approval for following instructions in a reasonable amount of time. Also, it might help to use mild nonphysical punishment, such as restriction of a privilege, for not following instructions.

A behavioral approach asks what the child *does* that's a problem and how the *consequences and circumstances* might be altered to change the child's behavior. Such an approach to treatment has been found highly effective by parents and teachers in many cases, if not most.[16]

Uses and Abuses of Medication

Any medication can be abused, but most people do not abuse drugs. In fact, any substance can be abused, although most people do not abuse the substances they use. The popular perception may well be that children are over-medicated and that psychoactive drugs prescribed for emotional and behavioral problems are abused in most instances. The reality is quite different.[17]

Medicine is regularly accepted by most people as help for a variety of diseases

> The popular perception may well be that children are over-medicated and that psychoactive drugs prescribed for emotional and behavioral problems are abused in most instances. The reality is quite different.

and disorders, but there is still considerable resistance to the notion that medication should be used for the emotional and behavioral disorders from which many children and adults suffer.[18] Moreover, although any medication can be abused, the benefits of psychoactive drugs far outweigh the dangers of abuse.

Evidence is accumulating that many or most emotional and behavioral disorders involve brain differences. Furthermore, many disorders, including some of the more common ones like ADHD, anxiety, depression, bipolar disorder, obsessive-compulsive disorder, and so on are usually responsive to medication, and drug therapies for them are often successful.[19] The large-scale study known as MTA (multi-modal treatment study of ADHD) found that medication alone produced significant improvement and better results than other therapy alone, although the best results were obtained with a combination of medication and social interventions.[20] The study involved multiple sites and very carefully monitored psychopharmacology (drug therapy). Good psychopharmacology, which too often is not practiced, involves careful monitoring of the effects of drugs, and it requires getting the right dosage of the right drug. Some drugs work better for some children than for others, but so far the only way to find out what drug works is to try one. Getting the dosage right, so that the child is neither under- nor over-medicated requires not only knowledge of drugs and dosage levels but careful monitoring of the effects at home and school.

Combined Treatments

The best results of treatment are almost always obtained by combining medication and cognitive-behavioral therapy (CBT). People do not need to choose between them—to choose only one or the other. Cognitive-behavioral therapy combines the behavioral approach with concern for the child's thinking and emotional reactions to things. Drugs can be used along with CBT. Most serious mental health problems, whether or not special education is part of the treatment, are best addressed through a combination of appropriate psychopharmacology, a behavioral program to address the "symptoms" or behavioral problem, and talking with the child about thoughts and feelings related to the problem and how to manage one's own behavior and feelings.

Failure to combine treatments into a multi-modal or multifaceted attack on the problem is usually a mistake. Drugs themselves may be of some help, but their effects are likely to be maximal only if parents and teachers are helped to see how they can manage the problem better. Behavior management alone is sometimes difficult or impossible until a prescription drug helps improve the child's behavior to the point that behavior therapy has a chance. Talk therapy alone is seldom enough, but talking with the child about the problem and its management is extremely important in a comprehensive approach. The talk need not be about unconscious or hidden motivations or feelings, but can be more productively focused on what the child did and include talking about very practical ways of helping oneself behave better. Finally, we note that the *talking should not occur while the child is misbehaving*, but soon after, when the incident is over and the child is calm. Talking to the child during misbehavior is likely to be unproductive and lead to arguing and exacerbation of the problem.

The MTA study found extremely good results from carefully administered, carefully monitored combined treatments. In fact, when good medication and good behavior therapy were combined, the children with ADHD did very well, were liked by other kids, and became very "normal" in their behavior.

School-Based Treatment

Making schools the central location for the treatment of children's mental health problems—school-based mental health services—is an idea that has prominent proponents.[21] However, as others have pointed out, there is no realistic hope (for a variety of reasons) that we will see a five-fold increase in the identification and treatment of children with EBD, either in special education or any other form of special service.[22]

> Making schools the central location for the treatment of children's mental health problems—school-based mental health services—is an idea that has prominent proponents.

True, only about one-fifth of a conservative estimate of the students who need treatment for EBD receive such services. The fact is that most students with EBD are now—and are extremely likely to remain—in general education. They are in ordinary classes in neighborhood schools with classroom teachers who have not been trained to be special educators. The data suggest that only the most severe cases of EBD are receiving special education now, and that is likely to continue to be the case.[23]

However, classroom teachers with little or no training as special educators can learn better behavior management strategies. Positive, supportive school-wide practices (often referred to as SWPBIS for school-wide positive behavioral interventions and supports) can make a significant difference in students' lives as well as in the emotional "climate" of the school. Positive intervention and support (PBIS) can help many youngsters whose emotional or behavioral problems make school particularly difficult for them, even if it's implemented in a specific classroom, not school-wide.[24]

PBIS is basically a behavioral approach to students' problems that puts the emphasis on positive behavior and support for the youngster. (It emphasizes incentives rather than punishment.) CBT and medication may also be part of the "package" of treatment, but the emphasis is on what teachers and other school staff can do to manage problem behavior in a more positive and supportive way.

Benefits of Treatment

The benefits of treatment may well be both a nearly immediate improvement in behavior and emotions and better long-term performance. Treatment should be not only about making things easier for the child or parents or teachers in the short run, but also about improving the child's prospects for the future. In school, this can mean greatly improved outcomes for the student's socialization, academic success, and graduation.

Treatment carries the possibility—indeed, a high probability—of improvement in behavior and mitigation of suffering. But effective treatment may also carry neurological benefits for the child. That is, CBT as well as medication may have the benefit of improving brain function.[25] It isn't helpful to let mental health problems go untreated, especially when effective treatment can potentially change lives immediately and well into the future.

> Treatment carries the possibility—indeed, a high probability—of improvement in behavior and mitigation of suffering.

Risks of Treatment

Treatment of any kind carries risks. There simply is no non-risk response to a problem. As we have discussed, one risk is stigma—the negative reaction of other people to the fact of treatment. Another risk is the possibility of misguided effort—maltreatment. Some forms of treatment may amount to quackery, to taking up time and money for worthless treatment. However, these risks pale in comparison to the possible benefits of competent treatment.

Treatment risk tends to be overestimated by many people. Fear of treatment and the stigma associated with it is often worse than the stigma itself. In fact obsession with stigma may make it worse, not only for the child receiving treatment but for others whose parents or teachers may be contemplating it.

Consequences of Nontreatment and Poor Treatment

As we mentioned earlier, most children with mental health difficulties receive no treatment at all. The probable consequences of such nontreatment are severe. Perhaps journalist Judith Warner has written most eloquently about what's at stake:

> The widespread, unthinking trivialization of mental health disorders in our public discourse isn't just hurtful and poisonous, however. It can even be dangerous for children with mental health issues, if it leads their parents to minimize their problems and not seek help for them. (And it does: Studies show that parents who don't believe that children's disorders are "real" don't get their kids help, even when the children are visibly showing symptoms.)[26]

The likelihood that nontreatment of mental health problems will result in the horrible acts of violence that are committed by those who are mentally ill is very small. That is, most people who are mentally ill do *not* inflict suffering on many others—they don't go berserk and kill or maim others or themselves. But they and their caretakers often suffer miserably for years, just as those with physical ailments may suffer and demand extraordinary care and sacrifice from their families.

> Clearly, the evidence is on the side of treatment. Nevertheless, nontreatment characterizes what we typically do now.

Clearly, the evidence is on the side of treatment. Nevertheless, nontreatment characterizes what we typically do now. The implementation of SWPBIS or even PBIS in specific classrooms would represent a significant advance in our responsiveness to mental health issues. We must not let the arguments against treatment continue to carry the day. The machismo tradition of toughing it out and going it alone must yield to the realization that accepting help is no shame. Obsession with shame and stigma and trying to avoid these problems merely creates an even greater social burden that is added to the suffering imposed by mental ill health. Treatment must be based on what's currently available and effective, not on what happened decades ago. And although the cost issue can't be avoided, the immediate cost of treatment must not be allowed to overshadow the long-term cost of ignoring problems.

All in all, we have a great deal to lose by nontreatment. The thing most likely to haunt us or lead our children to conclude that we made bad choices is our unwillingness to give treatment, our decision to do nothing or nothing much in response to mental health problems. The specter of inadequate treatment should trouble us. Poor treatment is tantamount to no treatment at all, and it can even make things worse instead of better. Good treatment takes time and money, and many citizens are reluctant to spend either—time or money. Too often, the treatment children receive is partial and inadequate (perhaps drugs alone, or too few sessions of CBT), often determined by attempts to control costs or satisfy insurance programs.

Too often, the public is short-sighted and cynical in its response to mental health issues. Sometimes, the professionals providing mental health services are incompetent. Sometimes they make claims of the effectiveness of their treatments that are unjustified, simply not supported by data related to best practices.

Finally, although we could immediately begin to do things that would be an improvement—like consistently using effective teaching and behavior management practices in our schools[27]—there is no immediate "fix" to the problem of effective treatment for children with mental health difficulties. Not only do we need qualified psychiatrists, psychologists, and teachers to provide better services to more children, but training such personnel requires the commitment of much money and many years. Then, paying them to provide the good services that will help kids as much as possible will require additional expenditures. The required training and therapies won't and can't, for the most part, be provided by private funds. Unfortunately, the required training and therapies would require a huge public investment in the futures of children.

The problem is complicated by the fact that the evidence will simply not support some of the therapies and teaching procedures favored by some practitioners—psychiatrists and psychologists, as well as teachers.[28] Movement toward evidence-based practices will surely result in some out-of-joint noses unless everything, regardless of its merit from a scientific point of view, is accepted as evidence. Moving toward a science of education is made particularly difficult by entrenched interests and belief systems that defy logic and careful analysis of empirical data. In psychiatry and related branches of medicine and psychology, too, we can find individuals who do not see the advantages of the scientific method and rely on unproven (from a scientific perspective) assertions, tradition, superstition, or folk wisdom. Many of these individuals speak and write with considerable authority and are loathe to give up ideas discredited by scientific data. This is most unfortunate, as it makes the scandalous neglect of children with mental health difficulties even more tragic because some of those who work with such children will not serve them well.

> If the problem of the neglect of children with mental health difficulties were easily solved, it would have been solved long ago.

A Plan of Action

If the problem of the neglect of children with mental health difficulties were easily solved, it would have been solved long ago. This is a "hard nut to crack," and it will take sustained, concerted effort to see substantial improvement. So, what specific action can people in various roles—educators, parents, voters, legislators, advocates, therapists—take? We suggest some things that people can do, but you should understand three points:

1. These are only *some* of the things that can be done. The list for people in all roles could be expanded.
2. Individuals often fill multiple roles (e.g., an individual might be identified as an educator, a voter, and an advocate).
3. The fact that someone is not in a role listed here (e.g., not a legislator) does not exclude them from taking an action listed for that role (e.g., a legislator who is not an educator could well encourage the use by educators of effective instruction).

For starters, here are some things we think people in various roles could and should do to move us toward recognition and help rather than neglect.

Educators

◆ Use and encourage others to use effective instruction in academics and social skills. Remember that good instruction minimizes students' behavior problems.
◆ Employ good behavior management procedures. Focus most of your attention on what you want, not what you don't want; learn to use positive behavioral support.
◆ Seek out training, help, and mentors for aspects of effective instruction and management that you may not understand.
◆ Do not hesitate to ask for the evaluation of any student you believe may have mental health issues. Having a student with a mental health disorder does not mean that you have failed as a teacher or administrator.
◆ Remember that providing special education in elementary school may serve as a protective factor for later difficulties.[29]
◆ Visit the special education program and become familiar with it.

Parents

◆ Use good behavior management procedures in your home with your child.
◆ Realize that having a child with mental health difficulties does not mean that you have been or are a bad parent.
◆ Recognize the reality that if your child needs help for a special problem there is no alternative to labeling the problem; help can't be given for an unspecified difficulty.

◆ Remember that providing special education in elementary school may serve as a protective factor for later difficulties.
◆ Visit the special education program and become familiar with what goes on there and why.
◆ Be an advocate for the most appropriate education of your child and others.

Voters

◆ Support candidates for public office at all levels who understand the need for expanding mental health services for youngsters with mental health issues, including special education.
◆ Ask candidates for public office as early as possible in their candidacy what they think about mental health services for children and youth.
◆ Encourage other voters to support candidates for public office who will work for the expansion of services for youngsters with mental health problems.

Legislators

◆ Think of the long-term effects when considering legislation, not only short-term consequences.
◆ Reject party-line responses to budget and service issues.
◆ Be willing to vote for the expenditures necessary to provide the level of service required to better meet the needs of children and youth with mental health problems.
◆ Don't be among those who "hack away" at special education, only to find that children with disabilities are the ones who suffer. [30]
◆ Talk to teachers and families who are dealing with mental health issues.

Advocates

◆ Help educate the general public about the need for additional mental health services, including special education, for youngsters with mental health problems. This may include writing letters to the editors of newspapers, writing blogs, and taking issues to your school board, community meetings, and local events.

◆ Support legislation and administrative action that improves the availability of services for young people with mental health difficulties.

◆ Argue for additional expenditure of public funds for children with mental health problems, pointing out the long-term savings that more readily available services will accomplish.

Physicians and Other Therapists (Including Special Educators)

◆ Use evidence-based practices only; do not rely on testimonials in selecting treatments for any disorders.

◆ Realize that academic and social success in school are critically important for students. Both academic and social skills are essential for long-term mental health.

◆ Develop a close personal connection to the youngster, based on building trust and expressing confidence in his or her strengths and competencies.

◆ Realize that the right medication at the right dosage can make life much better for the child and all who interact with him or her.

Notes

1. For example, see Eakman (1999).
2. Engelmann and Carnine (2011), Kauffman (2010, 2011).
3. Earley (2006), Powers (2017, Warner (2010).
4. Aviv (2011).
5. Earley (2006), Kauffman (2011, 2013), Powers (2017), Warner (2010). See also Kauffman (2014), Kauffman and Badar (2013), and Samuels (2018).
6. See Aviv (2011), Earley (2006), Powers (2017), Warner (2010).
7. E.g., Hakim (2011).
8. See Earley (2006), Powers (2017), Warner (2010).
9. E.g., Kauffman and Landrum (2018b), Kazdin (2008), Kerr and Nelson (2010), Landrum (2017), Walker et al. (2004)
10. Earley (2006), Powers (2017).
11. Wiley, Brigham, Kauffman, and Bogan (2013), Wiley, Kauffman, and Plageman (2014), Wiley and Siperstein (2011).
12. See Kendziora (2004) for a summary of such research.

13. Kendziora (2004, p. 342).

14. Landrum (2015), Kazdin and Weisz (2003), Morris and Mather (2008).

15. See Alberto and Troutman (2012), Kauffman and Landrum (2018b), Kazdin (2008), Kerr and Nelson (2010).

16. Kauffman and Landrum (2018b), Kauffman et al. (2017), Kazdin (2008), Kerr and Nelson (2010).

17. Warner (2010).

18. Forness and Kavale (2001), Warner (2010).

19. See Jamison (1995), Kauffman and Landrum (2018b), Warner (2010).

20. Jensen et al. (2001); see also Hallahan et al. (2018), Rooney (2017).

21. See Evans et al. (2007), Robinson (2004).

22. Lane et al. (2012).

23. Forness et al. (2012).

24. See Kauffman et al. (2017), Kerr and Nelson (2010); See also www.pbis.org/school/what_is_swpbs.aspx or do a web search for PBIS.

25. See Porto et al. (2009), Warner (2010).

26. Warner (2010, p. 192).

27. See Engelmann and Carnine (2011), Kauffman (2010, 2011), Kauffman and Brigham (2009).

28. See, for example, Kauffman (2010, 2011), Ruscio (2002), Specter (2007, 2009); see also Foxx and Mulick (2016).

29. Hart et al. (2017), Kauffman (2014).

30. Levy (2017).

7

What Educators Should Do First

We have additional suggestions for first responders, who are most likely to be teachers and others who work in schools. These suggestions go well beyond the more general ones we provided in Chapter 6. They are not detailed enough, however, to constitute a complete guide for practice. We cite other sources that provide additional, more detailed information about particular problems and practices. Our focus here is on teachers and what they could—and in our opinion *should* do—to help address the problem of neglect of students with mental health problems, likely to be called ED or some variant that represents the ED category of disability under IDEA. However, we also realize that *should* (or ought) implies *can*, and sometimes realities such as a particular class, parental prerogatives, administrative directions, laws, or regulations constrain what teachers *can* do (at least what is possible in a literal sense—or at least possible without getting fired).

We recommend trying to practice primary prevention whenever possible, so that behavior problems never occur at all. However, once someone sees a behavior problem and primary prevention isn't

> Once someone sees a behavior problem and primary prevention isn't possible for that student, secondary prevention is critically important.

possible for that student, secondary prevention is critically important. It's important to get on the problem as soon as possible (ASAP), to intervene as early as possible so that problems don't get any worse than necessary and might be reversed. So, although we believe that following our suggestions will help prevent many problems from showing up in the first place, they'll also help someone problem-solve, which is the essence of secondary prevention. If secondary prevention—getting on a problem quickly—isn't implemented, then the problem is likely to get to the point at which the objective is just to minimize the damage: tertiary prevention.

Make Instruction the Best It Can Be

We can't overemphasize the importance of getting instruction right. Good instruction is important in its own right, as many students with mental health problems have academic weaknesses.[1] Moreover, good instruction may keep lots of kids from misbehaving, simply because success in academics is highly gratifying. Academic struggles increase a student's irritability and tendency to engage in behavior that avoids academic tasks that are too difficult—or too easy, so that a student is tempted to misbehave out of boredom. So, make sure, first thing, that the problem is NOT a result of instruction that isn't right for the student in question. Of course, we need to get more specific about what we mean by "good instruction."[2] We have several suggestions for things teachers should think about, all of which are important. The order in which we discuss them isn't really indicative of their importance. The sequence is only important because the first letter of each key word (CLOCS-RAM) gives us a mnemonic—a memory device to help us remember what we consider the seven most important elements of good instruction.[3] Here are the elements: Clarity (of instructions), Level (of the task), Opportunity (to respond), Consequences (of performance), Sequence (of activities) + Relevance (of the task to the student's life), Application (to everyday life), and Monitoring (of performance).

> Good instruction isn't the only thing involved in behavior management, but it's the *first* thing a teacher should think about when behavior *is* a problem.

As we suggest later, good instruction isn't the only thing involved in behavior management, but it's the *first* thing a teacher should think about when behavior *is* a problem. In our opinion, the things we suggest about instruction apply in the general case, regardless of the student's age, grade, or culture. They are ways of practicing both primary and secondary prevention—helping to keep problems from developing and reducing problems we call EBD, even more generally "mental health problems."

Elements of Good Instruction

Clarity of Instructions

Trying to make instructions perfectly clear is an extremely important part of good teaching. A student should know, and be told if necessary, exactly what to do—what is expected academically *and* behaviorally. A teacher may easily fall into the trap of assuming that a student knows what to do when that student really doesn't. Sometimes, students misbehave because they don't know exactly what they're expected to do. And lots of times students who are problems just "don't get it" when others do. So, we suggest that giving instructions the best way requires thinking about making them as simple as possible. First, make sure the student is paying attention. It's good to have eye contact with the student if possible. Second, use really plain language (keep the instructions as simple as possible). Third, give only one instruction at a time, if possible, so that the student doesn't get confused. Sometimes, it's necessary to tell the student what to do in sequence (e.g., "first, hang up your coat, then get the things you need, and then sit down at your desk"), but it's always important to make the list as short and clear as possible. Fourth, give the student a few seconds to do what's expected when giving a direction about what the student is to do right away. Finally, follow through with consequences. Show clear approval for following directions. If the student has a choice, then follow through. For example, if you've said, "Either sit down now, or I'll call _____," then follow through by calling _____ if the student doesn't sit down within a few seconds. If the student does follow your direction to sit down, then immediately say something like, "I'm glad you chose to sit down."

Try to imagine what it's like to be the student who's listening to the instructions. Sometimes what seems really simple to us isn't simple to a student who's just learning something. It helps to imagine ourselves in a situation that's new to us, what it's like to be given instructions for something we've never done before. Often, the students we teach have never done what it is we are trying to teach them, so a student may really have only a vague notion of what we expect. Therefore, it's important to keep instructions simple, direct, and clear to make sure the student has plenty of time to follow them, and then to show approval for following them.

> It's important to keep instructions simple, direct, and clear to make sure the student has plenty of time to follow them, and then to show approval for following them.

Level of the Task

Some things are hard, and some are easy. But things are hard or easy only in a *relative* sense—harder for some of us than for others. It's just very, very frustrating to be in a situation in which most of the others "get it" and we don't. And when most of the others "get it" and we don't … well, we just want to be somewhere else. So, the point is, really, to make sure the level of the task fits the student, is something *that* student actually can do, isn't too hard and isn't too easy, either. Sure, we all want to be challenged, so a task can be too easy, too, and when that's the case we tend to get silly, not pay much attention, do things (sometimes inappropriate things) we wouldn't if the task were actually a challenge. If a task is too easy, we tend to see it as a waste of time. The students we teach aren't much different from us in that regard.

So, what percentage of correct responses gives us a clue that the task is too hard or too easy? Well, that depends on whether we're looking at correct responding when we're starting on something or when we think we're done teaching it. When we start to teach something, we'd expect less than 100% correct responding, and if we get that level of correctness right away, then we know the task is too easy. All correct—100%—is what we're hoping for after we've just taught something, because 100% shows clear mastery. But, in the beginning, when we're introducing a new task for the first time, then less than 70% correct shows that the task is too hard. Once we've taught something and

> Once we've taught something and then go back to it to review, we'd expect about 90% correct or higher if we've taught well.

then go back to it to review, we'd expect about 90% correct or higher if we've taught well.

Opportunities to Respond

Sometimes, students (including us adults) sit through what seem to be interminable sessions in which they're (or we're) bombarded with things from a speaker but never expected to respond, except perhaps with relief (or applause) at the end. Most adults are used to that sort of thing in religious services and lectures, but after about an hour we tend to get fidgety. Younger people tend to get fidgety after doing nothing in much less time. We've all heard the common complaint of children: "There's nothing to *doooooo!*"

Good lessons give the student lots of opportunities to *do* something, opportunities to answer or perform—to say or write or manipulate or construct something. Opportunity (or opportunities) to respond (OTR) is important, whether it is a particular student or the individual as part of a group that is responding. In other words, it's important for *each and every* student to have frequent OTR, which is not the case if the individual has only a single OTR per lesson.

Unfortunately, life in school too often involves mostly listening and waiting, not responding and getting feedback. There's an old saying, "Idle hands are the devil's workshop." It's not just hands but minds and mouths that need to be kept busy if students are to behave well. Planning lessons to engage students in responding takes a lot of time, but it's terribly important. The responding can be choral or group responding, but it's important to keep all students engaged as much as possible in writing, saying, giving hand signals, or otherwise *doing* something other than listening. This is important not only as a way of keeping students busy but as a way of knowing whether they are "getting" what it is we're trying to teach.

Consequences of Performance

Too often, students don't get feedback right away, one way or the other, about the correctness or desirability of what they've done. If they don't know or if they have to wait to find out, a lot of them lose interest, get confused, and just stop performing. Actually, we do the same kind of thing ourselves. The best instructors, whether they're school teachers, parents, or anyone else, let learners know right away whether they're right or wrong. They don't hesitate to tell you when you're wrong, but they're light on the criticism and emphasize getting things right rather than focusing on what's wrong. They're heavy on the praise for getting things right or doing what's expected. Those who are most successful with the greatest number of other people aren't stingy in showing approval.

Showing approval and giving encouragement are known technically as positive reinforcement *if the desired behavior increases*. Giving lots of positive reinforcement for the kind of performance you want is a critical aspect of good teaching, whether it's academic or social

> Giving lots of positive reinforcement for the kind of performance you want is a critical aspect of good teaching, whether it's academic or social behavior that's being taught.

behavior that's being taught. We all thrive on the praise and approval of people who are in control of important aspects of our lives, even if we sometimes act like we don't care.

Sequence of Activities

Lots of things that are relatively difficult for a student need to be broken down into steps, and these steps need to be taught in the right sequence. Sometimes, students don't succeed because they do things in the wrong order. So, when we're teaching something we need to be aware of what needs to be done first and then how the sequence goes. It's also critically important to make sure the student has the *prerequisite* skills. That is, it makes no sense to try to teach a sequence for which a student doesn't know an earlier step. This means that following a sequence in a specified curriculum is useless if the individual doesn't have the skills necessary to start the sequence. For some students, it's really important to get them

> Really good teaching involves thinking about the sequence for doing something that may seem automatic once the student gets the hang of it.

to slow down, do the first step, then the next, and so on. The task might seem easy to us, but it's not necessarily easy or intuitive to the student. Sometimes a "task analysis" is required—thinking about just how we do something, so that we can teach it step-by-step.

Really good teaching involves thinking about the sequence for doing something that may seem automatic once the student gets the hang of it. This kind of analysis is involved in *all* teaching, whether it is athletics, music, dance, and so on. It is necessary for good teaching of academics and social graces, too. Teaching things in sequence is very important, but so is getting the big idea. Ideally, the student sees the progression or framework leading to the more general skill we want them to learn.

Relevance of the Task to the Student

Being required to learn something just for the sake of learning it when we see no point in it makes us grumpy. This is why good teachers always try to find a way to make what they're teaching meaningful in some way to the student. Remember, too, that although a teacher may see the relevance of a task (for example, finding the area of a rectangle), the student may not. Sometimes, the matter of relevance is just a matter of making the task fun, a puzzle to be solved, a contest, or a race against time,

> Good teachers always try to find a way to make what they're teaching meaningful in some way to the student.

especially if what's being taught is really abstract. Things we do are sometimes only relevant to us because we make games of them.

Application to Everyday Life

One way of making something relevant to a student is applying the task to everyday life. Sometimes, this is a real stretch, especially when the task involves very abstract ideas or things that aren't part of everyday life in the student's culture. Sometimes, it's important to teach students skills that may open doors for them in the future and to emphasize future opportunities. Occasionally, what we want students to learn is a part of only a very few people's everyday life.

> Good teachers always try to find something that ties learning to the student's daily experience—or, at least, something the student has experienced or experiences once in a while or wants or may have the opportunity to do.

But good teachers always try to find something that ties learning to the student's daily experience—or, at least, something the student has experienced or experiences once in a while or wants or may have the opportunity to do. Moreover, we want students to be able to apply what they've learned to everyday problems, to learn a generalization rather than just an isolated concept or skill.

Monitoring Performance

Keeping track of how a student is performing really helps us teach better, and it helps us communicate better with others about just what the problem is, what we've tried, and how well it has worked. Sometimes, it's really important for the teacher to break measurement down into smaller units (like words read correctly per minute rather than paragraphs read correctly in a longer period of time). The usual standardized tests are given too infrequently and give the teacher information that is too general and too late to be of much benefit in instruction. For a student who has learning and behavior problems, it's necessary for the teacher to devise little, short, frequent tests or checks to see what that student has learned. Actually, little, short, frequent tests will help a teacher know more about the learning or performance of all students. Monitoring performance is also helpful to all students, and particularly helpful to some students. It helps them see their progress or regression and encourages them to do better. So, don't keep your monitoring to yourself. Share it with your students.

To reiterate, the teacher's first concern when any student is misbehaving, regardless of age or grade or culture, should be the *instruction* that student is receiving. We know that academic achievement is a weakness of many students with emotional and behavioral problems, and even if a student doesn't have a history of academic struggle or failure, instruction that is appropriate for him or her will lead to maximum academic success and decrease the tendency to misbehave.

The elements of good teaching we have mentioned apply in all cases. However, we do not explain here how *special* education is different from *general* education. Nor do we suggest elements of teaching particular subject matters (e.g., reading, social studies, science) that are important. We can suggest a few readings that might be helpful.[4]

Practice Other Good Behavior Management Strategies

We have already mentioned how important good instruction is in managing students' behavior. But, given that instruction is really good, there are other aspects of behavior management to be considered.

Some students exhibit unacceptable behavior even though they're getting good instruction. So, we are under no illusion that good instruction will solve *all* behavior problems. Good instruction is necessary, but it's not always sufficient. Therefore, we suggest a few fundamentals of behavior management here. For more information, you might turn to sources that discuss good behavior management in more detail.[5]

Elements of Good Behavior Management

Focus on What's Right, Not on What's Wrong

Perhaps it is impossible to overemphasize the importance of looking for and providing *positive consequences for appropriate behavior*. It is extremely important that the teacher or other adult know and make clear to the student what behavior is desirable *and* that such behavior will result in positive consequences. The positive consequence most important in teaching is teacher (and other adults') approval in the form of smiles, compliments, privileges, or other indications that good behavior has been noticed and that the teacher and other adults like it. Too often, the focus becomes what's wrong, but it should be on what's right. Peer attention and recognition of desirable behaviors are also important. Students need opportunities to give positive feedback to one another for improvements in performance or behavior.

> Perhaps it is impossible to overemphasize the importance of looking for and providing positive consequences for appropriate behavior.

Natural consequences should be used whenever possible. By "natural" we mean things that aren't contrived. Candies, points, and so on may be necessary sometimes, but teacher attention and praise or other signs of approval are more natural. Privileges in the classroom or school are also the "natural" consequences of good behavior.

Rewarding consequences should be as *immediate* as possible and should be given *frequently*. Adults tend to overestimate how frequently they show approval or otherwise reward desirable behavior with attention. They also tend to underestimate the importance of timing (i.e., providing *immediate* consequences). If a student is not behaving as well as expected, the immediacy and frequency of positive feedback are things to check and possibly adjust. It's not sufficient to assume that good behavior is its own reward or that the avoidance of criticism is enough to let the student know he or she is doing what's expected.

For more information on keeping punishment to a minimum and focusing on the positive, you might go to PBIS.org on the web. PBIS stands for *positive behavioral interventions and supports*, and although such procedures can be used with individuals in any setting it's possible to use this approach school-wide.

A widely used and excellent little book about behavior management includes a mnemonic about giving positive reinforcement: IFEED-AV.[6] The authors suggest that if someone wants to make positive feedback or reinforcement as effective as possible, then they should (we highlight the words in the mnemonic):

Give it as *Immediately* after desirable behavior as possible
Do so as *Frequently* as possible
Show Enthusiasm when giving it
Make *Eye contact* while doing it
Describe simply and clearly what the student has done to earn it
Build up *Anticipation* of earning it
Provide *Variety* in the reinforcement the student can earn.

When positive feedback or reinforcement doesn't seem to be working, it's usually because one or more of these things is inadequate. Usually, increasing the inadequate part of IFEED-AV will produce better results. The common complaint "I tried that, and it didn't work" is sometimes justified, but often the attempt to use positive reinforcement didn't work because one or more aspects of IFEED-AV were faulty.

Be Extremely Careful With Punishment

Punishment is dangerous, especially because it can easily be used unwisely or clumsily. Just because punishment has a long history of use in some cultures does not justify it.

> Punishment is dangerous, especially because it can easily be used unwisely or clumsily.

Furthermore, punishment is often addictive, in that it tends to have the appearance of "working" or having an immediate, desirable effect. When it is successful, its effects are immediate cessation of the punished behavior, which is highly rewarding to the person who administers the punishment, so they tend to use punishment more often. But in the long run, a focus on reward for desirable behavior is a much better choice.

It's not that punishment is *never* appropriate, but there are four things about punishment that we want to make clear:

1. Punishment should *never* involve hitting, humiliating, or in any other way being violent or abusive. If punishment is going to be used, it should involve nonviolent consequences, such as losing a privilege. It must be reasonable and understandable to the student (e.g., not involve threats the adult can't or won't make happen or something drastic, like losing a privilege for six months).

2. Punishment should be as immediate as possible, not long-delayed. Like rewarding or reinforcing consequences, immediacy is extremely important. Also, follow-through is extremely important, so that the punishment someone says *will* happen *does* happen.

3. Punishment should be clearly and easily avoidable by behaving appropriately. This also means that the student must know exactly what will be punished and exactly how to behave to obtain positive consequences instead.

4 Punishment must *not* be the primary focus of behavior management. The list of things that will be punished should be *very* short—way shorter than the list of things that will be rewarded with praise, approval, attention, or privileges. The focus should be on what the student *should* do, on what is desired and appropriate.

Try keeping track of the ratio of positive to negative consequences. Positive ought to outnumber negative consequences by a ratio of at least 5:1. Remember, *punishment alone is a dead end; it is not sufficient to produce desirable conduct.* Remember also that teachers, parents, and other adults should emphasize desirable behavior, not merely harp on misbehavior. Lecturing, sarcasm, and corporal punishment must be studiously avoided.

Try the Simplest Things First

Many classroom behavior problems are complex and don't have a simple solution. Nevertheless, simple things like clear, consistent instructions or examples (showing—providing a model) sometimes quickly and effectively resolve seemingly intransigent problems.

Relatively sophisticated or technical information is readily available about behavior management, so it's easy to forget that simple, direct approaches can be effective. Simple things save time and energy, at least when they work, and little time and energy are lost if they don't. So, they're almost always worth trying.

Simple isn't the same as simplistic, and we don't want to suggest oversimplified approaches that have been discredited or are unethical—things like threats, lecturing, sarcasm, or corporal punishment. Simple things may seem obvious to somebody who's taking a fresh look at a situation, but they're easy to overlook when you're the teacher responsible for managing a difficult child or class. So, this question is always worth asking: Have I overlooked something that's really easy, simple and ethical that might work? And this question is worth asking, too: If I *have* tried a simple thing that didn't seem to work, have I implemented it well and consistently?

Simple things that might work, especially if they're done really well, include telling (giving instructions), showing (providing examples), and giving choices. We include considerations for each of these and provide an example of a simple but effective behavior management strategy that one teacher tried.

> Simple things that might work, especially if they're done really well, include telling (giving instructions), showing (providing examples), and giving choices.

Instructions

When a student either does things he or she shouldn't or fails to do what's desired, the simplest, most direct approach may be using *instructions*—telling the student exactly and clearly what's expected. You may at first think that this approach is unrealistic because the student has obviously been told how to behave. However, there are lots of ways to make instructions *in*effective, including using too many words—verbal clutter. Use as few words as possible to convey the idea. Give the instructions in a clear, firm, non-tentative but polite and non-angry way. Make sure you have the student's attention before you give the instruction, and make sure you give only one instruction at a time. Wait a reasonable amount of time for the student to comply, and monitor whether the student is doing as told. Make sure you express approval when the student complies with your instruction.

Examples

Good examples or models are simple but indispensable tools in teaching. It's easy to forget that the social skills that seem to be second nature to most of us are unfamiliar, even mysterious, to some youngsters. "You need to pay attention" may mean little or nothing to many students with serious attention problems. In teaching students to pay attention to their work it might be necessary to (1) demonstrate for them the way they behave when they're *not* paying attention (e.g., looking around the room, playing with an object), (2) model for them the kind of behavior involved in paying attention (e.g., reading, writing answers, looking at the teacher when the teacher is talking), and (3) have them practice the behavior involved in paying attention and give them feedback on their performance. Being polite, sharing, waiting your turn, and so on, are examples of other types of behavior that some students may not understand without being shown examples. Make sure you give both correct and incorrect examples, and make sure to tell the student what's an incorrect and what's a correct example. Give the student feedback, especially positive feedback for correct behavior, when he or she tries to imitate the examples you show.

Choices

Most people become resentful of not having choices about things. Most of us behave badly when we feel "boxed in" by having no choice. Students usually like being able to choose certain features of their instruction or classroom environment. The savvy teacher is careful about the choices students are allowed to make for themselves. Inventive teachers can usually find alternatives to nearly any assignment, all of which have instructional value, and allow a difficult student to choose the one he or she prefers.

Too few choices often lead to resentment and resistance to authority. Too many choices can leave a person frustrated and unable to make a decision. For obvious reasons, sometimes a teacher *shouldn't* allow a student to have a choice because we know that in some situations a student is highly likely to make a very bad choice. Master teachers understand that choices have to be structured to prevent catastrophic consequences and to promote personal responsibility.

In structuring choices for students, make sure to do these things: First, look for appropriate options for the student. Second, make sure you can be happy with the choice a student makes. Third, make sure the choices a student has are consistent with that student's developmental level.

We said we'd give an example of a teacher finding a simple, straightforward solution to a behavior problem. Here's an example from the literature on behavior management.[7]

> I was teaching sixth-graders who ate lunch in my classroom, bringing their lunch trays back to the classroom from the cafeteria. When they finished their lunches, the routine was that they scraped their trays into a waste can in the hallway and stacked their trays on a rack. I thought the rule was clear, that no more than four students were to be in the hallway at the same time. However, I had a lot of difficulty with too many kids going out to scrape their trays at the same time. And if five or six of my students got out into the hallway at the same time, they started horsing around, shoving, pushing, doing gross things with the leftovers, and things like that. They were noisy, and what they did often led to other problems like teasing, threatening, spilling food, and getting food on their clothes. Finally, it occurred to me that what might work was some sort of "pass" that would make the rule easier to monitor, something tangible that would regulate the traffic. So, I got four short pieces of bamboo that students could use as "batons" or passes. Then the rule became, "You may go out to scrape your tray *only* if you have a baton." Actually, the students saw it as a sort of fun game of passing the baton to the next person of their choosing. It did occur to me that this could have created problems, but for this group it worked. The students could have started doing bad things with the batons. We could have had fights and teasing and hard feelings over who got the baton next, and other things could have gone wrong, too. But those bad things didn't happen. And if things had gone wrong, I wouldn't have lost much, if anything, by trying. I learned that sometimes little gimmicks work, especially in regulating turns or movement. After all, why do you suppose some stores have customers take a number so they know when it's their turn to be waited on?

Be Proactive

One helpful way of thinking how misbehavior gets started and what can be done about it is the "acting out cycle."[8] The beginning phases in the cycle are called "calm," "trigger," "agitation," and "acceleration."

> Adults should take the initiative to interact in a positive and supportive way with students before troublesome behavior gets started.

Calm

All students are sometimes calm, meaning that they aren't engaged in any kind of maladaptive behavior. It's critically important to pay attention to and interact positively with them when they are so. In fact, adults should take the initiative to interact in a positive and supportive way with students *before* troublesome behavior gets started. For example, a teacher might comment positively on some aspect of the student (grooming, clothing, activity) while the student is calm (behaving appropriately). Remember IFEED-AV and the elements of positive reinforcement that make it work best, then look for opportunities to reinforce calm behavior.

Trigger

A trigger is something that sets someone off. It refers to some incident or circumstance that sets the occasion for troublesome behavior because it upsets an individual's feeling of calmness. It could be an interaction or other event such as being teased, hearing a disparaging remark, encountering a particular person, or encountering a particular demand or expectation. Regardless of what it is, it's important to know that it upsets the student's calm behavior and that needs to be resolved. Just making sure the student knows that you understand the discomfort, anxiety, frustration, or anger about the trigger may help. But it is also important to help the student solve the problem. You may be able to come up with ways of solving the problem, but the idea of dealing with triggers is to teach the *student* to solve the problem by himself or herself. An unresolved problem often leads to agitation.

Agitation

Usually, you'll see signs that a trigger has occurred, even if you don't know exactly what it is. Agitation is usually signaled by a noticeable change in behavior—a marked increase or decrease in activity. This might take the form of very frequent movement from one group to another, repetition of words or phrases that aren't conversational, or other repetitive behavior like tapping or rocking. Or it might be indicated by staring, mumbling, or otherwise having a rigid posture or showing signs of social withdrawal. Usually, the student who is agitated has difficulty staying on task and concentrating. A student who is agitated can easily become involved in acceleration, so it's a good idea to help the student learn ways of returning to calmness.

Acceleration

In the acceleration phase, a student gets involved in a struggle with someone. That is, the student looks for opportunities, and typically finds one, to engage someone in a back-and-forth such as questioning and arguing or taunting and challenging. The "my turn–your turn" or back-and-forth can involve anyone, but the teacher is a prime target for engagement. Usually, it becomes a battle of wills. The best thing to do when a student is in the acceleration phase is just refuse to be drawn in, to decline getting involved in an argument or struggle. Showing your own agitation (and agitated feelings are understandable) by doing things like making challenging or demeaning remarks, grabbing the student, or lecturing are going to be unproductive. We do not suggest how to handle an out-of-control student here, but the wise teacher plans ahead and is ready to state calmly an expectation and consequence if the student doesn't comply with the direction (e.g., "You need to sit down now, or I'll call your mother."). It's really important not to state a consequence on which you can't follow through and actually do it. Also, it's important to state the expectation clearly and only once, to give the student a few seconds to comply, and to follow through with the stated consequence if the student does not comply.

Pay Attention to Little Things—*ONLY IF, They Are Precursors of Serious Problems*

By the time a student's behavior is far down this chain of acting-out stages, it is too late to take the best proactive action. The key is intervening early in the chain—starting with paying attention to the calm stage. The most successful teachers are those who are sensitive to the first indications of problems and intervene early in the chain or cycle to stop them. They recognize the earliest, often subtle signs that a student is beginning to go "off track." They do not let these little things grow into big problems. They may seem to the untrained and inexperienced to be intolerant or obsessive, but they understand how seemingly insignificant behavior grows into serious problems. For example, a teacher might understand how a seemingly innocuous teasing word or gesture can quickly lead to a behavioral upset or confrontation. Therefore, he or she may intervene early and subtly to put a stop to something with the potential to lead to serious misconduct.

Lots of professional literature about behavior management recommends ignoring the little things—what we might call "trash" behavior. Ignoring things that don't matter is good advice. Teachers and other adults should not be distracted by and waste time on trivia. That is, they should not waste time and energy on little things that might be irritating but don't present any real danger. They shouldn't get involved in negative interactions with students over things that don't matter. Rather, they should focus on the positive behavior that's desirable. Focusing on positive consequences for desirable behavior is much more productive.

However, it's also important *not* to ignore the little things that *are* important precursors—*likely to lead to bigger problems*.[9] This is often a difficult distinction to make. The only way to know what's likely to lead to bigger problems is to learn through careful observation what usually leads up to big problems. Remember this about prevention: No one can prevent something that's already happened. Someone can prevent only what they anticipate. So, it's really important to be aware of the signs and signals that something worse is likely to happen *if* a given behavior is ignored.

Do Not Hesitate Unnecessarily to Refer a Student for Evaluation

We suggest that doing the things we mentioned previously *before* referral will prevent many problems from occurring at all. However, if a teacher has practiced the foregoing suggestions faithfully but a student is still exhibiting problematic behavior, we recommend referral for evaluation to see whether the student qualifies for special education. Referring a student for evaluation for possible special education is required by law for any student suspected of having a disability related to mental health.[10]

One reason we suggest that teachers should not hesitate to ask for the evaluation of any student they believe may have mental health problems has to do with the feeling of failure on the part of educators. Having a student who has mental health difficulties does *not* mean that a teacher or administrator has failed. In fact, we suggest that a major problem is failure to recognize immediately enough that a student has emotional or behavioral problems that might constitute a disorder. Early intervention and prevention are not compatible with allowing identification of problems to be blocked by competing concerns, as we noted in Chapter 5.

Our comments from this point on are directed to classroom teachers, as they are the most obvious first responders in a school. The reasons for referring a student for evaluation and possible special education or other mental health service are to get help for the student and yourself as the student's teacher. This can't be done well without spending time and energy thinking and writing clearly about the problems and your concerns.

> Referring a student for evaluation for possible special education is required by law for any student suspected of having a disability related to mental health.

Referring a student for evaluation initiates what can be a difficult process, and it has its costs and risks. It is not something that should be done needlessly, but it is also not something that should be delayed when the student has responded unsatisfactorily to good teaching and behavior management. Usually, a referral is made to a school psychologist or administrator. Sometimes, it is made to an interdisciplinary team. The student should be tested and observed, and a team of individuals will determine whether the student does or does not qualify for special education. Some referrals are better than others. Here, we suggest the major features of good referrals.

Elements of a Good Referral

Clear Description of the Problem or Issue

It won't be enough to describe the problem in only general terms, such as "He is often noncompliant" or "She sasses me." You need to give examples of specific behavior and, if possible, include times, places, and circumstances that apply. If possible, define and count the behavior you define so that you can quantify the problem.

For example, you might be able to include in your referral something like "He often threatens, tries to harm, or hits other students in the class. I have kept a record of this kind of behavior for the past three weeks, and he did this 43 times. His threats include menacing gestures like shaking his fist or saying things like 'You've got an appointment with this (showing his fist).' I heard him tell another boy in the class, 'You do, and I'll kill you' while glowering at him. On October 13, as he was leaving the class, I saw him hit a girl in the back for no apparent reason. The next morning, October 14, he accused another boy of saying something he didn't like and punched him hard in the chest (I did not hear what the boy said). On October 15, I saw him deliberately trip another student by putting his foot out as the other student walked by." The more explicit and specific you can be, the better.

Specification of Exactly What Has Been Done

One thing that is sure to delay evaluation of a student is lack of clarity in describing what you have done as a teacher to avoid problems. The people who get your referral will need to know exactly what you have done to try to avert problems. In addition to describing your use of the teaching and management suggestions we have provided, you might describe exactly what you have done to deal with the problem behavior.

Documentation of Involvement of Parents

Referral of a student should not come as a surprise to parents. They should know that you are making the referral and why you are concerned. It's important that they be involved every step of the way and that you document how you have involved them. So, you should communicate your concerns to parents from the first time you observe the problem behavior. You should keep careful records of the dates and communications you have with parents so that the people reading your referral know what you have done and that the parents are not in the dark about the problem.

Expression of Concerns

The people who read your referral should know precisely what you are concerned about and why. The student's future is not the only legitimate concern you may have. You may also express concern for your ability to give other students in the class what they need or to express concern for the safety or learning of other students.

Final Comments

Students whose problems are primarily externalizing—acting out or hyper-aggressive, for example—are seldom overlooked by teachers. We recommend paying careful attention also to internalizing emotional and behavioral problems, such as depression, self-deprecation, and feelings of worthlessness or hopelessness. Remember, too, that some youngsters both externalize and internalize problems. Be especially watchful for signs of possible suicide, such as feelings of worthlessness and hopelessness or talk of suicide. Don't hesitate to refer a student for mental health consultation or counseling if you see any sign that leads you to suspect a student might be suicidal.

Reversing the neglect of youngsters' mental health and special education needs that has become so characteristic of our society will not be easy. It will require the concerted action of many people. Perhaps it must start with first responders, including teachers, who are in the best position to see that a student's emotions and behavior are unlike those of most other students and take appropriate action. Although special education is often misunderstood, and too many politicians and others may continue to "hack away" at it,[11] early special education may well help prevent later difficulties or make them more treatable.[12]

We close with a reiteration of the scandalous neglect of children's mental health and the importance of schools in providing mental health services, including special education, to children who need them.

> Reversing the neglect of youngsters' mental health and special education needs that has become so characteristic of our society will not be easy.

Approximately 80% of children who need mental health services do not receive them, with even higher rates of unmet need among Latino populations and the uninsured (Kataoka, Zhang, & Wells, 2002). The most common disorders among youth are depression, anxiety disorders, oppositional defiant disorder, conduct disorder, and attention-deficit/hyperactivity disorder (ADHD).... However, to expand the focus beyond diagnosable mental disorders, even larger numbers of young people (over 20% of youth) experience psychosocial problems and/or impairments that place them at risk for negative outcomes in adulthood.... Schools provided 70–80% of the services to children and adolescents who received any services, and for the majority of those students this was their only source of care.[13]

By adolescence, approximately 30% to 40% of youth in the United States will have been diagnosed with at least 1 mental disorder.... Left untreated, mental disorders first appearing during the elementary school years tend to persist.... [L]ess than half of affected youth receive mental health care ... [and] racial and ethnic minority children receive fewer and poorer-quality mental health services.... [E]ducators and school staff have assumed frontline mental health provider roles for affected children, with more than half the youth who seek services receiving them in school-based settings.[14]

Notes

1. Kauffman and Landrum (2018b), Mattison and Blader (2013).
2. We've extracted what we consider to be good teaching from the research and practice guidelines suggested by, among others, the following: Bateman (2004), Carnine, Silbert, Kame'enui and Tarver (2005, 2010), Coyne, Kame'enui and Carnine (2006), Engelmann (1997), Engelmann and Carnine (2011), Hirsch, Lloyd, and Kennedy (2014), Landrum, Wiley, Tankersley, and Kauffman (2014), Nelson, Benner, and Bohaty (2014), Rosenshine (2008), and Walker et al. (2004).
3. This mnemonic device and description of good teaching were suggested by Kauffman et al. (2011).
4. For more on how special and general education are different, see Kauffman (2015), Kauffman et al. (2018), Pullen and Hallahan (2015), Zigmond and Kloo (2017). For more suggestions about teaching in general, see Hirsch et al. (2014), Nelson et al. (2014), Nicholson (2014); see also references in note 2 above. For more on teaching specific subject matter, see Pullen and Cash (2017) for reading, Troia, Graham, and Harris (2017) for writing, Fuchs,

Malone, Seethaler, Powell, and Fuchs (2017) for arithmetic, and Scruggs, Mastropieri, Brigham, and Milman (2017) for science and social studies.

5. For more details about principles of behavior management, you might turn to books like the following: Alberto and Troutman (2012), Garner et al. (2014), Kauffman and Landrum (2018b), Kauffman et al. (2011), Kerr and Nelson (2010); Rhode, Jenson, and Reavis (2010), Walker et al. (2004), Walker and Gresham (2014).

6. Rhode et al. (2010).

7. This is based on a case described in Kauffman et al. (2011). See also Kauffman, Pullen, and Akers (1986).

8. The acting out cycle was described by Colvin, Sugai, and Patching (1993) and later elaborated by Colvin (2004).

9. See Smith and Churchill (2002).

10. See Bateman (2007, 2017), Huefner and Herr (2012), Martin (2013), Yell (2012), Yell et al. (2017).

11. Levy (2017).

12. Dunlap and Fox (2014), Hart et al. (2017), Strain, Barton, and Bovey (2014), Walker et al. (2014).

13. Evans, Rybak et al. (2014, p. 394).

14. Sanchez, Comacchio, Poznanski, Golik, Chou, and Comer (2018, p. 153).

References

Abernathy, G. (2017, September 22). Trump's supporters *are* normal. *The Washington Post*, A17.

Achenbach, J., & Nutt, A. E. (2016, August 16). Donald Trump and a personality disorder that's all about him ... or you. *Washington Post*, E5.

Alberto, P. A., & Troutman, A. C. (2012). *Applied behavior analysis for teachers* (9th ed.). Upper Saddle River, NJ: Pearson.

Alexander, F. G., & Selsnick, S. T. (1966). *The history of psychiatry: An evaluation of psychiatric thought from prehistoric times to the present.* New York: Harper & Row.

Alexandrova, A. (2017, October 7). *Does anyone know what mental health is?* Oxford University Press (OUPblog). Retrieved on October 8, 2017 from https://blog.oup.com/2017/10/mental-health-philosophy/?utm_source=feedblitz&utm_medium=FeedBlitzRss&utm_campaign=oupblog

American Psychiatric Association. (2013). *Diagnostic and statistical manual* (5th ed.). New York: Author.

Anastasiou, D., Gregory, M., & Kauffman, J. M. (in press Commentary on Article 24 of the CRPD: The right to education. In I. Bantekas, M. Stein, & D. Anastasiou (Eds.), *Commentary on the UN Convention on the Rights of Persons with Disabilities.* New York, NY: Oxford University Press.

Anastasiou, D., & Kauffman, J. M. (2010). Disability as cultural difference: Implications for special education. *Remedial and Special Education, 33*, 139–149. doi:10.1177/0741932510383163.

Anastasiou, D., & Kauffman, J. M. (2013). The social model of disability: Dichotomy between impairment and disability. *Journal of Medicine and Philosophy, 38*, 441–459.

Anastasiou, D., & Kauffman, J. M. (2011). A social constructionist approach to disability: Implications for special education. *Exceptional Children, 77*, 367–384. Reprinted in A. R. Sadovnik, P. W Cookson, S. F. Semel, & R. W Coughlan (Eds.) (2018). *Exploring education: An introduction to the foundations of education* (5th ed.) (pp. 554–579). New York: Routledge.

Anastasiou, D., Morgan, P. L., Farkas, G., & Wiley, A. (2017). Minority disproportionate representation in special education: Politics and evidence, issues and implications. In J. M. Kauffman & D. P. Hallahan (Eds.), *Handbook of special education* (2nd ed., pp. 897–910). New York: Routledge.

Aviv, R. (2011, May 30). God knows where I am: What should happen when patients reject their diagnosis? *The New Yorker*, 56–65.

Bateman, B. D. (2004). *Elements of successful teaching: A best practices handbook for beginning teachers.* Verona, WI: Attainment.

Bateman, B. D. (2007). Law and the conceptual foundations of special education practice. In J. B. Crockett, M. M. Gerber, & T. J. Landrum (Eds.), *Achieving the radical reform of special education: Essays in honor of James M. Kauffman* (pp. 95–114). Mahwah, NJ: Lawrence Erlbaum Associates.

Bateman, B. D. (2017). Individual education programs for children with disabilities. In J. M. Kauffman, D. P. Hallahan, & P. C. Pullen (Eds.), *Handbook of special education* (2nd ed., pp. 87–104). New York: Taylor & Francis.

Bayat, M. (2011). Clarifying issues regarding the use of praise with young children. *Topics in Early Childhood Special Education, 31,* 121–128.

Bower, E. M. (1960). *Early identification of emotionally handicapped children in school.* Springfield, IL: Thomas.

Burns, B. J., Costello, E. J., Angold, A., Tweed, D., Stangl, D., Farmer, E. M. Z., & Erkanli, A. (1995). DataWatch: Children's mental health service use across service sectors. *Health Affairs, 14,* 147–159.

Carnine, D. W., Silbert, J., Kame'enui, E. J., & Tarver, S. G. (2005). *Teaching struggling and at-risk readers: A direct instruction approach.* Upper Saddle River, NJ: Merrill Prentice-Hall.

Carnine, D. W., Silbert, J., Kame'enui, E. J., & Tarver, S. G. (2010). *Direct instruction reading* (5th ed.). Upper Saddle River, NJ: Merrill Prentice-Hall.

Carrero, K. M., Collins, L. W., & Lusk, M. E. (2017). Equity in the evidence base: Demographic sampling in intervention research for students with emotional and behavioral disorders. *Behavioral Disorders, 43,* 253–261.

Centers for Disease Control and Prevention (2013, May 17). *Mental health surveillance among children—United States, 2005–2011.* Retrieved on May 30, 2013 from www.cdc.gov/mmwr/preview/mmwrhtml/su6202a1.htm?s_cid=su6202a1_w.

Colvin, G. (2004). *Managing the cycle of acting-out behavior in the classroom.* Eugene, OR: Behavior Associates.

Colvin, G., Sugai, G., & Patching, B. (1993). Pre-correction: An instructional approach for managing predictable problem behaviors. *Intervention in School and Clinic, 28,* 143–150.

Conduct Problems Prevention Research Group. (2011). The effects of the fast track preventive intervention on the development of conduct disorder across childhood. *Child Development, 82,* 331–345.

Cook, B. G., & Ruhaak, A. E. (2014). Causality and emotional or behavioral disorders: An introduction. In P. Garner, J. M. Kauffman, & J. G. Elliott (Eds.), *The Sage handbook of emotional and behavioral difficulties* (2nd ed., pp. 97–108). London: Sage.

Costello, E. J., Egger, H., & Angold, A. (2005). 1-year research update review: The epidemiology of child and adolescent psychiatric disorders: I. Methods and public health burden. *Journal of the American Academy of Child and Adolescent Psychiatry, 44,* 972–986.

Coyne, M. D., Kame'enui, E. J., & Carnine, D. W. (2006). *Effective teaching strategies that accommodate diverse learners* (3rd ed.). Upper Saddle River, NJ: Merrill Prentice Hall.

Dionne, E. J. (2016, October 6). How Trump corrupts the GOP. *Washington Post,* A19.

Dionne, E. J., Mann, T. E., & Orenstein, N. J. (2017, September 24). How Trump is helping to save our democracy. *Washington Post,* B5, B5.

Donovan, M. S., & Cross, C. T. (Eds.). (2002). *Minority students in special and gifted education.* Washington, DC: National Academy Press.

Duncan, B. B., Forness, S. R., & Hartsough, C. (1995). Students identified as seriously emotionally disturbed day treatment: Cognitive, psychiatric, and special education characteristics. *Behavioral Disorders, 20,* 238–252.

Dunlap, G., & Fox, L. (2014). Supportive interventions for young children with social, emotional, and behavioral delays and disorders. In H. M. Walker & F. M. Gresham (Eds.), *Handbook of evidence-based practices for emotional and behavioral disorders: Applications in schools* (pp. 503–517). New York: Guilford.

Dunlap, G., Strain, P. S., Fox, L., Carta, J. J., Conroy, M., Smith, B. J., et al. (2006). Prevention and intervention with young children's challenging behavior: Perspectives regarding current knowledge. *Behavioral Disorders, 32,* 29–45.

Eakman, B. K. (1999, October). No: Don't give educational experts another tool to 'psychologize' the school curriculum. *Insight,* 41, 43.

Earley, P. (2006). *Crazy: A father's search through America's mental health madness.* New York: Penguin.

Engelmann, S. (1997). Theory of mastery and acceleration. In J. W. Lloyd, E. J. Kameenui, & D. Chard (Eds.), *Issues in educating students with disabilities* (pp. 177–195). Mahwah, NJ: Erlbaum.

Engelmann, S., & Carnine, D. (2011). *Could John Stuart Mill have saved our schools?* Verona, WI: Attainment.

Evans, S. W., Rybak, T., Strickland, H., & Owens, J. S. (2014). The role of school mental health models in preventing and addressing children's emotional and behavioral problems. In H. M. Walker & F. M. Gresham (Eds.), *Handbook of evidence-based practices for emotional and behavioral disorders: Applications in schools* (pp. 394–409). New York: Guilford.

Evans, S. W., Weist, M. D., & Zewelanji, N. S. (Eds.). (2007). *Advances in school-based mental health interventions: Best practices and program models. Volume II.* Kingston, NJ: Civic Research Institute.

Fisher, M. (2016, October 23). Trumpism isn't going away: Has the Republican nominee transformed America, or simply revealed it? *Washington Post,* A1, A4.

Forness, S. R., Freeman, S. F. N., Paparella, T., Kauffman, J. M., & Walker, H. M. (2012). Special education implications of point and cumulative prevalence for children with emotional or behavioral disorders. *Journal of Emotional and Behavioral Disorders,* 20, 1–14.

Forness, S. R., & Kavale, K. A. (2001). Ignoring the odds: Hazards of not adding the new medical model to special education decisions. *Behavioral Disorders,* 26, 269–281.

Forness, S. R., & Knitzer, J. (1992). A new proposed definition and terminology to replace "serious emotional disturbance" in Individuals With Disabilities Education Act. *School Psychology Review,* 21, 12–20.

Forness, S. R., Walker, H. M., & Serna, L. A. (2014). Establishing an evidence base: Lessons learned from implementing randomized controlled trials for behavioral and pharmacological interventions. In H. M. Walker & F. M. Gresham (Eds.), *Handbook of evidence-based practices for emotional and behavioral disorders: Applications in schools* (pp. 567–582). New York: Guilford.

Foxx, R. M., & Mulick, J. A. (Eds.). (2016). *Controversial therapies for autism and intellectual disabilities: Fad, fashion, and science in professional practice* (2nd ed.). New York: Francis & Taylor.

Franken, A. (2017). *Al Franken: Giant of the Senate.* New York: Twelve.

Fuchs, L. S., Malone, A. S., Seethaler, P. M., Powell, S. R., & Fuchs, D. (2017). Intervention to improve arithmetic, word-problem, and fraction performance in students with mathematics disabilities. In J. M. Kauffman, D. P. Hallahan, & P. C. Pullen (Eds.), *Handbook of special education* (2nd ed., pp. 558–570). New York: Taylor & Francis.

Garner, P., Kauffman, J. M., & Elliott, J. G. (Eds.). (2014). *The Sage handbook of emotional and behavioral difficulties* (2nd ed.). London: Sage.

Gordon, N. (2017, September 20). *Race, poverty, and interpreting overrepresentation in special education.* Washington, DC: Brookings Institution. Retrieved on September 23, 2017 from www.brookings. edu/research/race-poverty-and-interpreting-overrepresentation-in-special-education/

Grigorenko, E. L. (2014). Genetic causes and correlates of EBD: A snapshot in time and space. In P. Garner, J. M. Kauffman, & J. G. Elliott (Eds.), *The Sage handbook of emotional and behavioral difficulties* (2nd ed., pp. 131–144). London: Sage.

Hakim, D. (2011, June 6). A disabled boy's death, and a troubled system. *The New York Times*, A1, A14–15.

Hallahan, D. P., Kauffman, J. M., & Pullen, P. C. (2018). *Exceptional learners: An introduction to special education* (14th ed.). Upper Saddle River, NJ: Pearson Education.

Hallenbeck, B. A., & Kauffman, J. M. (1995). How does observational learning affect the behavior of students with emotional or behavioral disorders? A review of research. *Journal of Special Education, 29*, 45–71. doi: 10.1177/00224669950290010

Harris, E. A. (2017, October 28). At a troubled school, another tale of bullying: Former student says he tried suicide. *New York Times*, A17.

Harry, B., & Klingner, J. (2007). Discarding the deficit model. *Educational Leadership, 64*(5), 16–21.

Harry, B., & Klingner, J. (2014). *Why are so many minority students in special education? Understanding race & disability in schools* (2nd ed.). New York: Teachers College Press.

Hart, S. R., Musci, R. J., Slemrod, T., Flitsch, E., & Ialongo, N. (2017, October 2). A longitudinal, latent class growth analysis of the association of aggression and special education in an urban sample. *Contemporary School Psychology.* Retrieved on November 11, 2017 from https://link.springer.com/article/10.1007/s40688-017-0160-z

Hirsch, S. E., Lloyd, J. W., & Kennedy, M. J. (2014). Improving behavior through instructional practices for students with high incidence disabilities: EBD, ADHD, and LD. In P. Garner, J. M. Kauffman, & J. G. Elliott (Eds.), *The Sage handbook of emotional and behavioral difficulties* (2nd ed., pp. 205–220). London: Sage.

Hobbs, N. (1974). Nicholas Hobbs. In J. M. Kauffman & C. D. Lewis (Eds.), *Teaching children with behavior disorders: Personal perspectives* (pp. 142–167). Upper Saddle River, NJ: Merrill/Prentice Hall.

Huefner, D. S., & Herr, C. M. (2012). *Navigating special education law and policy.* Verona, WI: Attainment.

Imray, P., & Colley, A. (2017). *Inclusion is dead: Long live inclusion.* New York: Routledge.

Jamison, K. R. (1995). *An unquiet mind.* New York: Knopf.

Jensen, P. S., Hinshaw, S. P., Swanson, J. M., Greenhill, L. L., Conners, C., Arnold, L., et al. (2001). Findings from the NIMH Multimodal Treatment Study of ADHD (MTA): Implications and applications for primary care providers. *Journal of Developmental & Behavioral Pediatrics, 22,* 60–73.

Johnson, W., Turkheimer, E., Gottesman, I. I., & Bouchard, T. J., Jr. (2009). Beyond heritability: Twin studies in behavioral research. *Current Directions in Psychological Science, 18,* 217–220.

Julien, M. (2014). *The only girl in the world: A memoir.* New York: Little, Brown.

Kagan, R. (2016, August 3). There is something wrong with Donald Trump. *Washington Post,* A 17.

Karp, S. (2017, October 16). *WBEZ investigation: CPS secretly overhauled special education at students' expense.* Retrieved on October 18, 2018 from www.wbez.org/shows/wbez-news/wbez-investigation-cps-secretly-overhauled-special-education-at-students-expense/2f6907ea-6ad2-4557-9a03-7da60710f8f9

Kataoka, S. H., Zhang, L., & Wells, K. B. (2002). Unmet need for mental health care among U. S. children: Variation by ethnicity and insurance status. *American Journal of Psychiatry, 159,* 1548–1555.

Kauffman, J. M. (1976). Nineteenth-century views of children's behavior disorders: Historical contributions and continuing issues. *Journal of Special Education, 10,* 335–349.

Kauffman, J. M. (1999). How we prevent the prevention of emotional and behavioral disorders. *Exceptional Children, 65,* 448–468.

Kauffman, J. M. (2007). Conceptual models and the future of special education. *Education and Treatment of Children, 30,* 241–258.

Kauffman, J. M. (2008). Would we recognize progress if we saw it? A commentary. *Journal of Behavioral Education, 17,* 128–143.

Kauffman, J. M. (2009). Attributions of malice to special education policy and practice. In T. E. Scruggs & M. A. Mastropieri (Eds.), *Advances in learning and behavioral disabilities: Volume 22. Policy and practice* (pp. 33–66) Oxford, UK: Elsevier.

Kauffman, J. M. (2010). *The tragicomedy of public education: Laughing and crying, thinking and fixing.* Verona, WI: Attainment.

Kauffman, J. M. (2011). *Toward a science of education: The battle between rogue and real science.* Verona, WI: Attainment.

Kauffman, J. M. (2013). Labeling and categorizing children and youth with emotional and behavioral disorders in the USA: Current practices and conceptual problems. In T. Cole, H. Daniels, & J. Visser (Eds.), *International companion to emotional and behavioural difficulties.* London: Routledge.

Kauffman, J. M. (2014). How we prevent the prevention of emotional and behavioral difficulties in education. In P. Garner, J. M. Kauffman, & J. G. Elliott (Eds.), *The Sage handbook of emotional and behavioral difficulties* (2nd ed., pp. 505–516). London: Sage.

Kauffman, J. M. (2015). Why we should have special education. In B. Bateman, M. Tankersley, & J. Lloyd (Eds.), *Enduring issues in special education: Personal* perspectives (pp. 397–408). New York: Routledge.

Kauffman, J. M., & Anastasiou, D. (in press). On cultural politics in special education: Is much of it justifiable? *Journal of Disability Policy Studies.*

Kauffman, J. M., Anastasiou, D., Badar, J., & Hallenbeck, B. A. (in press). Becoming your own worst enemy: Converging paths. In C. Boyle, S. Mavropoulou, J. Anderson, & A. Page (Eds.), *Inclusive education: Global issues & controversies.* Rotterdam, Netherlands: SENSE.

Kauffman, J. M., Anastasiou, D., Badar, J., Travers, T. C., & Wiley, A. L. (2016). Inclusive education moving forward. In J. P. Bakken & F. E. Obiakor (Eds.), *Advances in special education, Volume 32: General and special education in an age of change: Roles of professionals involved* (pp. 153–177). Bingley, UK: Emerald.

Kauffman, J. M., & Badar, J. (2013). How we might make special education for students with emotional or behavioral disorders less stigmatizing. *Behavioral Disorders, 39,* 16–27.

Kauffman, J. M., & Badar, J. (2014). Instruction, not inclusion, should be the central issue in special education: An alternative view from the USA. *Journal of International Special Needs Education, 17,* 13–20.

Kauffman, J. M., & Badar, J. (2016). It's instruction over place—not the other way around! *Phi Delta Kappan, 98*(4), 55–59.

Kauffman, J. M., & Badar, J. (2018). Extremism and disability chic. *Exceptionality, 26,* 46–61. First published online, March 1, 2017. doi :10.1080/09362835.2017.1283632

Kauffman, J. M., Bantz, J., & McCullough, J. (2002). Separate and better: A special public school class for students with emotional and behavioral disorders. *Exceptionality, 10,* 149–170. doi:10.1207/S15327035EX1003_1

Kauffman, J. M., & Brigham, F. J. (2009). *Working with troubled children.* Verona, WI: Attainment.

Kauffman, J. M., Conroy, M., Gardner, R., & Oswald, D. (2008). Cultural sensitivity in the application of behavior principles to education. *Education and Treatment of Children, 31,* 239–262. doi:10.1353/etc.0.0019

Kauffman, J. M., Felder, M., Ahrbeck, B., Badar, J., & Schneiders, K. (in press). Inclusion of *all* students in general education? International appeal for a more temperate approach to inclusion. *Journal of International Special Needs Education.*

Kauffman, J. M., Hallahan, D. P., Pullen, P. C., & Badar, J. (2018). *Special education: What it is and why we need it* (2nd ed.) New York: Routledge.

Kauffman, J. M., Nelson, C. M., Simpson, R. L., & Ward, D. R. (2017). Contemporary issues. In J. M. Kauffman, D. P. Hallahan, & P. C. Pullen (Eds.), *Handbook of special education* (2nd ed.) (pp. 16–28). New York: Taylor & Francis.

Kauffman, J. M., & Landrum, T. J. (2006). *Children and youth with emotional and behavioral disorders: A history of their education.* Austin, TX: Pro-Ed.

Kauffman, J. M., & Landrum, T. J. (2018a). *Cases in emotional and behavioral disorders of children and youth* (4th ed.). Upper Saddle River, NJ: Prentice Hall.

Kauffman, J. M., & Landrum, T. J. (2018b). *Characteristics of emotional and behavioral disorders of children and youth* (11th ed.). Upper Saddle River, NJ: Pearson Education.

Kauffman, J. M., & Lloyd, J. W. (2017). Statistics, data, and special education decisions: Basic links to realities. In J. M. Kauffman, D. P. Hallahan, & P. C. Pullen (Eds.), *Handbook of special education* (2nd ed., pp. 29–39). New York: Taylor & Francis.

Kauffman, J. M., Lloyd, J. W., Baker, J., & Riedel, T. M. (1995). Inclusion of all students with emotional or behavioral disorders? Let's think again. *Phi Delta Kappan, 76,* 542–546.

Kauffman, J. M., Mock, D. R., & Simpson, R. L. (2007). Problems related to underservice of students with emotional or behavioral disorders. *Behavioral Disorders, 33,* 43–57.

Kauffman, J. M., Pullen, P. L., & Akers, E. D. (1986). Classroom management: Teacher-child-peer relationships. *Focus on Exceptional Children, 19*(1), 1–10.

Kauffman, J. M., Pullen, P. L., Mostert, M. P., & Trent, S. C. (2011). *Managing classroom behavior: A reflective case-based approach* (5th ed.) Upper Saddle River, NJ: Pearson Education.

Kauffman, J. M., Simpson, R. L., & Mock, D. R. (2009). Problems related to underservice: A rejoinder. *Behavioral Disorders, 34,* 172–180.

Kazdin, A. E. (2008). *The Kazdin method for parenting the defiant child.* Boston: Houghton Mifflin.

Kazdin, A. E., & Weisz, J. R. (Eds.). (2003). *Evidence-based psychotherapies for children and adolescents.* New York: Guilford.

Kendziora, K. T. (2004). Early intervention for emotional and behavioral disorders. In R. B. Rutherford, M. M. Quinn, & S. R. Mathur (Eds.). *Handbook of research in emotional and behavioral disorders* (pp. 327–351). New York: Guilford.

Kerr, M. M., & Nelson, C. M. (2010). *Strategies for addressing behavior problems in the classroom* (6th ed.). Upper Saddle River, NJ: Merrill Prentice Hall.

Kessler, R. C., Chiu, W. T., Demler, O., & Walters, E. E. (2005). Prevalence, severity, and comorbidity of 12-month DSM-IV disorders in the national comorbidity survey replication. *Archives of General Psychiatry, 62,* 617–627.

Konopasek, D. E., & Forness, S. R. (2014). Issues and criteria for effective use of psychopharmacological interventions in schooling. In H. M. Walker & F. M. Gresham (Eds.), *Handbook of evidence-based practices for emotional and behavioral disorders: Applications in schools* (pp. 457–472). New York: Guilford.

Lambros, K. M., Ward, S. L., Bocian, K. M., MacMillan, D. L., & Gresham, F. M. (1998). Behavioral profiles of children at-risk for emotional and behavioral disorders: Implications for assessment and classification. *Focus on Exceptional Children, 30*(5), 1–16.

Landrum, T. J. (2015). Science matters in special education. In B. Bateman, J. W. Lloyd, & M. Tankersley (Eds.), *Enduring issues in special education: Personal perspectives* (pp. 429–440). New York: Routledge.

Landrum, T. J. (2017). Emotional and behavioral disorders. In J. M. Kauffman, D. P. Hallahan, & P. C. Pullen (Eds.), *Handbook of special education* (2nd ed., pp. 312–324). New York: Routledge.

Landrum, T. J., Wiley, A. L., Tankersley, M., & Kauffman, J. M. (2014). Is EBD 'special', and is 'special education' an appropriate response? In P. Garner, J. M. Kauffman, & J. G. Elliott (Eds.), *The Sage handbook of emotional and behavioral difficulties* (2nd ed., pp. 69–81). London: Sage.

Lane, K. L., Kalberg, J. R., & Menzies, H. M. (2009). *Developing schoolwide programs to prevent and manage problem behaviors: A step-by-step approach.* New York: Guilford.

Lane, K. L., & Menzies, H. M. (Eds.). (2010). Special issue: Reading and writing interventions for students with and at risk for emotional and behavioral disorders. *Behavioral Disorders, 35*(2).

Lane, K. L., Menzies, H. M., Oakes, W. P., & Kalberg, J. R. (2012). *Systematic screenings of behavior to support instruction: From preschool to high school.* New York: Guilford.

Levy, L. (2017, October 30). *Why do politicians feel free to hack away at special education?* Retrieved on November 11, 2017 from www. huffingtonpost.com/entry/why-do-politicians-feel-free-to-hack-away-at-special_us_59f73bace4b05f0ade1b58c1

Lewis, M. (2017). *The undoing project: A friendship that changed our minds.* New York: Norton.

Lozada, C. (2017, September 24). Is Trump mentally ill? Or is America? Psychiatrists analyze the president and the politics that created him. *Washington Post,* B1, B5.

Martin, E. W., Jr. (2013). *Breakthrough: Federal special education legislation 1965–1981.* Sarasota, FL: Bardolf.

Mattison, R. E. (2014). The interface between child psychiatry and special education in the treatment of students with emotional/behavioral disorders in school settings. In H. M. Walker & F. M.

Gresham (Eds.), *Handbook of evidence-based practices for emotional and behavioral disorders: Applications in schools* (pp. 104–126). New York: Guilford.

Mattison, R. J., & Blader, J. C. (2013). What affects academic functioning in secondary special education students with serious emotional and/or behavioral problems? *Behavioral Disorders, 38*, 201–211.

McCrummen, S. (2014, November 1). A father's scars: For Va.'s Creigh Deeds, tragedy brings unending questions. *Washington Post*, A1.

Morris, R. J., & Mather, N. (Eds.). (2008). *Evidence-based interventions for students with learning and behavioral challenges*. Mahwah, NJ: Lawrence Erlbaum Associates.

Moyer, M. W. (2017). Journey to gunland. *Scientific American, 317*(4), 54–63.

National Mental Health Association. (1986). *Severely emotionally disturbed children: Improving services under Education of the Handicapped Act (P.L. 94–142)*. Washington, DC: Author.

Nelson, J. R., Benner, G. J., & Bohaty, J. (2014). Addressing the academic problems and challenges of EBD students. In H. M. Walker & F. M. Gresham (Eds.), *Handbook of evidence-based practices for emotional and behavioral disorders: Applications in schools* (pp. 363–377). New York: Guilford.

Nicholson, T. (2014). Academic achievement and behavior. In P. Garner, J. M. Kauffman, & J. G. Elliott (Eds.), *The Sage handbook of emotional and behavioral difficulties* (2nd ed., pp. 177–188). London: Sage.

Porto, P. R., Oliveira, L., Mari, J., Volchan, E., Figueira, I., & Ventura, P. (2009). Does cognitive behavioral therapy change the brain? A systematic review of neuroimaging in anxiety disorders. *Journal of Neuropsychiatry and Clinical Neurosciences, 21*, 114–125.

Powers, R. (2017). *No one cares about crazy people; The chaos and heartbreak of mental health in America*. New York: Hachette.

Pullen, P. C., & Cash, D. B. (2017). Reading. In J. M. Kauffman, D. P. Hallahan, & P. C. Pullen (Eds.), *Handbook of special education* (2nd ed., pp. 523–536). New York: Taylor & Francis.

Pullen, P. C., & Hallahan, D. P. (2015). What is special education instruction? In B. Bateman, J. W. Lloyd, & M. Tankersley (Eds.), *Enduring issues in special education: Personal perspectives* (pp. 37–50). New York: Routledge.

Reinke, W. M., Frey, A. J., Herman, K. C., & Thompson, C. V. (2014). Improving engagement and implementation of interventions for children with emotional and behavioral disorders in home and school settings. In. H. M. Walker & F. M. Gresham (Eds.), *Handbook of evidence-based practices for emotional and behavioral disorders: Applications in schools* (pp. 432–445). New York: Guilford.

Reisman, J. M. (1976). *A history of clinical psychology* (enlarged ed.). New York: Irvington.

Rhode, G., Jenson, W. R., & Reavis, H. K. (2010). *The tough kid book: Practical classroom management strategies* (2nd ed.). Eugene, OR: Pacific Northwest Publishing.

Robinson, K. E. (Ed.). (2004). *Advances in school-based mental health interventions: Best practices and program models. Volume I*. Kingston, NJ: Civic Research Institute.

Rooney, K. J. (2017). Attention-deficit/hyperactivity disorder. In J. M. Kauffman, D. P. Hallahan, & P. C. Pullen (Eds.), *Handbook of special education* (2nd ed., pp. 300–311). New York: Taylor & Francis.

Rosenshine, B. (2008). Systematic instruction. In T. L. Good (Ed.), *21st Century education: A reference handbook: Volume 1* (pp. 235–243). Thousand Oaks, CA: Sage.

Rubin, R. A., & Balow, B. (1978). Prevalence of teacher identified behavior problems: A longitudinal study. *Exceptional Children, 45*, 102–111.

Ruscio, J. (2002). *Clear thinking with psychology: Separating sense from nonsense.* Pacific Grove, CA: Wadsworth.

Samuels, C. A. (2018, March 19). Students with emotional disabilities: Facts about this vulnerable population. *Education Week.* Downloaded March 19, 2018 from https://www.edweek.org/ew/articles/2018/03/21/students-with-emotional-disabilities-facts-about-this.html?cmp=eml-enl-eu-news2-rm&M=58419997&U=1788915&print=1

Sanchez, A. L., Comacchio, D., Poznanski, B., Golik, A. M., Chou, T., & Comer, J. S. (2018). The effectiveness of school-based mental health services for elementary-aged children: A meta-analysis. *Journal of the American Academy of Child & Adolescent Psychiatry, 57*(3), 153–165.

Schaaff. S. V. (2016, November 1). Help is scarce for troubled youth: Even those whose need for psychiatric care is clear often go untreated. *Washington Post*, E1, E4.

Scruggs, T. E., Mastropieri, M. A., Brigham, F. J., & Milman, L. M. (2017). Science and social studies. In J. M. Kauffman, D. P.

Hallahan, & P. C. Pullen (Eds.), *Handbook of special education* (2nd ed., pp. 571–585). New York: Taylor & Francis.

Scull, A. (2015). *Madness in civilization: A cultural history of insanity from the Bible to Freud, from the madhouse to modern medicine.* Princeton, NJ: Princeton University Press.

Shaffer, D., Fisher, P., Dulcan, M. K., Davies, M., Piacentini, J., Schwab-Stone, M. E., et al. (1996). The NIMH Diagnostic Interview Schedule for Children Version 2.3 (DISC-2.3): Description, acceptability, prevalence rates, and performance in the MECA study. *Journal of the American Academy of Child and Adolescent Psychiatry, 35,* 865–877.

Shermer, M. (2017, November). *Mass public shootings & gun violence: Part I.* Retrieved on November 15, 2017 from youtube.com/watch?time_continue=2&v=yrK0excqg00

Smith, R. G., & Churchill, R. M. (2002). Identification of environmental determinants of behavior disorders through functional analysis of precursor behavior. *Journal of Applied Behavior Analysis, 35,* 125–136.

Specter, M. (2007, March 12). Annals of science. The denialists: The dangerous attacks on the consensus about H.I.V. and AIDS. *The New Yorker,* 32–38.

Specter, M. (2009). *Denialism: How irrational thinking hinders scientific progress, harms the planet, and threatens our lives.* New York: Penguin.

Strain, P. S., Barton, E. E., & Bovey, E. H. (2014). Evidence-based practices for infants and toddlers with autism spectrum disorders. (2014). In. H. M. Walker & F. M. Gresham (Eds.), *Handbook of evidence-based practices for emotional and behavioral disorders: Applications in schools* (pp. 475–502). New York: Guilford.

Sullivan, A. L. (2017). Wading through quicksand: Making sense of minority disproportionality in identification of emotional disturbance. *Behavioral Disorders, 43,* 244–252.

Tallent, G. (2017). *My absolute darling: A novel.* New York: Riverhead.

Troia, G. A., Graham, S., & Harris, K. R. (2017). Writing and students with language and learning disabilities. In J. M. Kauffman, D. P. Hallahan, & P. C. Pullen (Eds.), *Handbook of special education* (2nd ed., pp. 537–557). New York: Taylor & Francis.

Tucker, J. E. (2010–2011, Winter). "Child First" campaign. *The Maryland Bulletin, 81*(2), 3. Retrieved on May 17, 2011 from www.msd.edu/mdb/v131i2_1011_win.pdf.

U. S. Department of Health and Human Services. (2000). *Report of the Surgeon General's conference on children's mental health: A national action agenda*. Washington, DC: Author. (Note: This report may be found on line by going to www.ncbi.nlm.nih.gov. Start by searching for NBK44233, then click on NLM Catalog under Literature, then on Electronic Links.)

Walker, H. M., & Gresham, F. M. (Eds.). (2014). *Handbook of evidence-based practices for emotional and behavioral disorders: Applications in schools*. New York: Guilford.

Walker, H. M., Ramsey, E., & Gresham, F. M. (2004). *Antisocial behavior in school: Strategies and best practices* (2nd ed.). Pacific Grove, CA: Brooks/Cole.

Walker, H. M., Severson, H. H., Seeley, J. R., Feil, E. G., Small, J., Golly, A., et al. (2014). The evidence base for the First Step to Success early intervention for preventing emerging antisocial behavior patterns. In. H. M. Walker & F. M. Gresham (Eds.), *Handbook of evidence-based practices for emotional and behavioral disorders: Applications in schools* (pp. 518–533). New York: Guilford.

Wang, P. S., Berglund, P., Olfson, M., Pincus, H. A., Wells, K. B., & Kessler, R. C. (2005). Failure and delay in initial treatment contact after first onset of mental disorders in the national comorbidity survey replication. *Archives of General Psychiatry, 62*, 603–613.

Warner, J. (2010). *We've got issues: Children and parents in the age of medication*. New York: Riverhead Books.

Webster, D., Vernick, J., Crifasi, C., & McGinty, B. (2017, October 8). Five myths: Gun violence. *Washington Post*, B2.

Wiley, A L., Brigham, F. J., Kauffman, J. M., & Bogan, J. E. (2013). Disproportionate poverty, conservatism, and the disproportionate identification of minority students with emotional and behavioral disorders. *Education and Treatment of Children, 36*(4), 29–50.

Wiley, A. L., Kauffman, J. M., & Plageman, K. (2014). Conservatism and the under-identification of students with emotional and behavioral disorders in special education. *Exceptionality, 22*, 237–251.

Wiley, A. L., & Siperstein, G. N. (2011). Seeing red, feeling blue: The impact of state political leaning on state identification rates for emotional disturbance. *Behavioral Disorders, 36*, 195–207.

Wilson, P., & Frances, A. (2017, June). *Misdiagnosing Trump: Doc-to-doc With Allen Frances, MD*. Retrieved on November 11, 2017 from www.medpagetoday.com/psychiatry/generalpsychiatry/67728

Yell, M. L. (2012). *The law and special education* (3rd ed.). Upper Saddle River, NJ: Pearson.

Yell, M. L., Katsiyannis, A., & Bradley, M. R. (2017). The Individuals with Disabilities Education Act: The evolution of special education law. In J. M. Kauffman, D. P. Hallahan, & P. C. Pullen (Eds.), *Handbook of special education* (2nd ed., pp. 55–70). New York: Routledge.

Zigmond, N. P., & Kloo, A. (2017). General and special education are (and should be) different. In J. M. Kauffman, D. P. Hallahan, & P. C. Pullen (Eds.), *Handbook of special education* (2nd ed., pp. 249–262). New York: Routledge.

For Product Safety Concerns and Information please contact our EU
representative GPSR@taylorandfrancis.com
Taylor & Francis Verlag GmbH, Kaufingerstraße 24, 80331 München, Germany